IMPROVE YOUR SIGHT NATURALLY

PRICE 6op NET

IMPROVE YOUR SIGHT NATURALLY
Simple Rules for Better Vision

by

C. LESLIE THOMSON

of the Kingston Clinic, Edinburgh;
Director of Studies, Edinburgh School
of Natural Therapeutics

Illustrations by the Author

THORSONS PUBLISHERS LTD.
37/38 MARGARET STREET, LONDON, W.1

First published September 1956
as *Your Sight*
This Edition, revised and reset, September 1971

To
"GANNY"

ISBN 0 7225 0171 4

MADE AND PRINTED IN GREAT BRITAIN BY
MORRISON AND GIBB LIMITED, LONDON AND EDINBURGH

PREFACE

Our senses are classically considered to be five in number, each possessing a clearly defined function. On closer study, however, we find that this is an underestimate, and that the distinction between one sense and another is not always clear. Also, any sense is usually efficient only when it co-operates with one or more others.

Thus an impression which appears to arrive solely through one sense organ may, on analysis, be identified as a group of several different impressions arriving simultaneously and blended by the brain into a single perception.

How and why perceptions take the form they do is an entertaining rather than profitable field for speculation. All our sensations arrive at the brain in the form of tiny currents flowing through minute nerve fibres. Why, then, should a musical note normally register in our consciousness as something totally different from the taste of a pear, or the colour of a rose ? The ultimate mechanism which converts these electrical impulses into distinct mental impressions, and from these builds up what we call *perception*, is something which one may safely describe as totally insoluble. We may be able to trace the " wiring " and identify the " switchboards," but the human mind cannot really comprehend itself.

The workings of the simpler, more mechanical parts of the actual sense organ can, however, be fairly well understood. It is with these that we are principally concerned in this book—their method of function, and the physical and chemical circumstances which affect their ability to initiate accurate nerve currents. We shall also discuss the essential importance of rapid and accurate interpretation of these signals by the brain, and the factors which play upon this alertness of mind.

Most of us consider eyesight our most valuable sense, and, indeed, much of what we consider modern civilisation is based upon our ability to know where things are and something of their character, without touching them. It is also complementary to other senses in an almost incredibly complete way. For instance, a speaker may mumble a word or two, so that the listener is unable to hear the message clearly, but the listener's eye can note the movements of the speaker's mouth, his facial expression and even his hands, and so fill in the gaps. The listener may be quite unaware of the part played by vision—he only knows that the total impression was enough to convey the message satisfactorily.

Increasingly, the interdependence of one sense upon another is being recognised by those who study their workings. Unhappily, in many cases this realisation leads only to a multiplication of the number of specialists called upon when a person seeks to remedy a defect. As with other organs and parts of the body, what is really required is less specialisation, and a wider understanding of the patient's way of living and states of general health and mental outlook.

The essence of Nature Cure is the knowledge that the human body is a complete organism, with full powers of maintenance and self-repair. It requires only a modest supply of genuine raw materials, and reasonable handling by the owner. Given these, it will keep itself in full running order, with all faculties alert, throughout a long and active life. But because of its very completeness, any disturbance of the general balance is bound to affect every component part. Similarly, distress in any part affects the whole.

In any case of defective eyesight, therefore, the primary essential is to restore the balance of the body's supplies, and make more normal and reasonable the way in which the body is used.

In the following pages are described general and local attentions by which derangements of the supply systems and deficiencies of the eyes may be remedied and these organs brought to their most healthful and efficient state.

CHAPTER I

THE EYE

EVERYONE interested in maintaining or improving eyesight should bear in mind that the eyes are living organs, and integral parts of the body. Although this may seem an obvious suggestion, it is too often forgotten that these organs must be properly nourished and regularly exercised if they are to maintain their efficiency. Also, like every other part of the body, they are sensitive to the state of the individual's health, respond to emotional and physical strains, and, above all, are self-healing.

It is in the acceptance and logical application of such facts that the Nature Cure system of treatment differs so markedly from the orthodox.

The eye is composed of living cells, each dependent upon the bloodstream for its nourishment, oxygenation and cleansing. If the bloodstream is imperfect in any way, the cells will sooner or later show the effects of malnutrition, lack of oxygen or toxic overload. The nervous system controls the activities of the cells, regulates the flow of blood and blood fluids through the tissues, and maintains a constant watch on the state of the cells. Clearly, then, any variation in the blood composition is likely to alter the characteristics of the cells, and distress in the nervous system as a whole will be reflected in their activities.

The eye is a complex organ and, with its associated equipment, consists of a large number of different types of tissue, all interconnected. Vision can only function efficiently when these structures are able to co-operate fully. The general bodily condition may be such that one or other of the tissues is more affected than the rest, since each requires its own particular materials, but usually there is a lowering of efficiency in all parts when the health is poor.

It is generally true that the most highly developed structures and faculties are the first to be affected by conditions of ill-health. So it is that in most people visual efficiency is noticeably and rapidly lowered by difficult physical conditions. In special cases, however, the eyes may appear to be little affected even when other organs and tissues are seriously upset. This seems to occur principally in those whose livelihood is dependent upon good eyesight. In such circumstances, the intelligence of the system appears to arrange that so far as possible the eyes are maintained in good order, even at the expense of vital organs.

Smoking Detrimental

On the other hand, there are some factors which have a universally damaging effect. Tobacco, for example, is always detrimental to the eyesight, and in even moderate smokers the ability to distinguish colours is impaired.

Incidentally, it would appear reasonable to deduce at least a partial connection between the ten times greater incidence of colour-blindness in men than in women and the relative popularity of smoking in the two sexes.

While true colour-blindness is due to the absence or non-functioning of certain retinal cells, in many cases a reduced ability to differentiate colours can be caused by drugs, or even by general ill-health.

Although tobacco-smoke does irritate the eyeball

directly—as most non-smokers in cinemas and theatres know to their cost—the real harm to the sight is produced by the drug-effect within the blood.[1] Accordingly we consider Edgar Wallace's device of protecting his eyes by means of a very long cigarette-holder was based on a misunderstanding.

Far from possessing an immunity from such effects, the really healthy person is much more noticeably affected by the intake of a drug than is the unhealthy individual. Although to some this may seem paradoxical, the explanation lies in the higher standards attained in the healthy body and the correspondingly greater intolerance to impurities and poisons. When one realises that, with most drugs, what are called the " effects " are really the *defensive* acts of the body, it will be readily appreciated that the more healthy and vigorous the system, the more violent the response. In some cases, the less noticeable reaction of the unhealthy individual is simply a matter of proportion. If the subject's blood already has a high toxic content, the addition of a few extra grains of poison is scarcely noticed by the nervous sentinels, and accordingly little or no reaction occurs. The damaging effect of the drug, however, is just as serious, although it may take longer to show superficially.

To emphasise the living nature of the eye, it may be helpful to note a parallel in a more obvious member of the body. If we wish to possess a strong, useful arm, we know that it must be employed actively—exercised. We also know from experience that exercise movements must be intelligently selected. Restricted actions, if

[1] See *Why Not Smoke ?*

frequently repeated, tend to diminish the arm's useful range of movement. Heavy, slow exercise tends to produce large, slow-moving muscles. Light, quick and varied movements regularly carried to their limits, result in a limb which is mobile, responsive, and able to exert sustained effort over long periods of time without undue fatigue. And so it is with the eye. If asked to perform only a restricted range of actions, and seldom faced with unusual tasks, it slowly becomes less elastic, less adaptable, and too easily tired.

Eye Movements

Let us see how this applies to a common type of eye action—the process of reading. In this the eye is required only to move sufficiently to scan a line of type. In intensive reading this action may be repeated many thousands of times per day, and there is a serious possibility that the eye may gradually lose—through disuse—the ability to perform wider and more unusual movement. In reading there is a further restrictive effect, since the muscles which move the eye from left to right, and back again, are working fairly vigorously, while those which bring the eye slowly down the page are doing relatively little. The most probable result is that the muscles in the first group will become more quickly tired than the comparatively inert muscles of the second group. All these muscles are attached to the eyeball, and surround it closely. Since the eyeball is elastic any abnormal and uneven tension in the muscles tends to produce distortion, so that the spherical shape is lost, and the eyeball becomes somewhat flattened. Such a change produces imperfect focusing, and consequently the individual finds reading both tiring and difficult.

But there is one very important consideration : no matter how great the tendency for a bad habit to produce abnormality of this kind, so long as the individual's health is good, his eyes will remain unharmed even after long and repeated spells of difficult work.

Only when the health is poor, and the nutrition and nervous controls of the visual mechanism inadequate, is there any rapid breakdown or disorganisation of the sight. In health, the intelligence of the cells and the alertness of central controls prevent either damaging tensions or nutritional failure. In health, too, the body automatically exercises and keeps alert any muscles or other mobile tissues which might otherwise remain over-quiescent. When a potentially harmful situation arises, the part will become " fidgety " or painful, and the individual will more or less unconsciously take the proper steps to rectify the condition. In an unhealthy person the sentinels are less alert, and all manner of abuse is permitted to continue without rousing the safety devices into action.

As already mentioned, the eye is a very highly developed sense organ. The Nature Cure practitioner believes that many bodily abnormalities may produce distress or disturbance in any such organ. This is in contrast to those specialists who even at the present day appear to believe that the cause of any distress must lie either within the particular organ affected, or in a germ. Increasingly, the damaging effects of both common and " wonder " drugs are being recognised, but the similar effects of wrong living are less readily acknowledged.

Before turning to practical matters, let us first deal with a few elementary yet essential theoretical points about the eye and its mode of action.

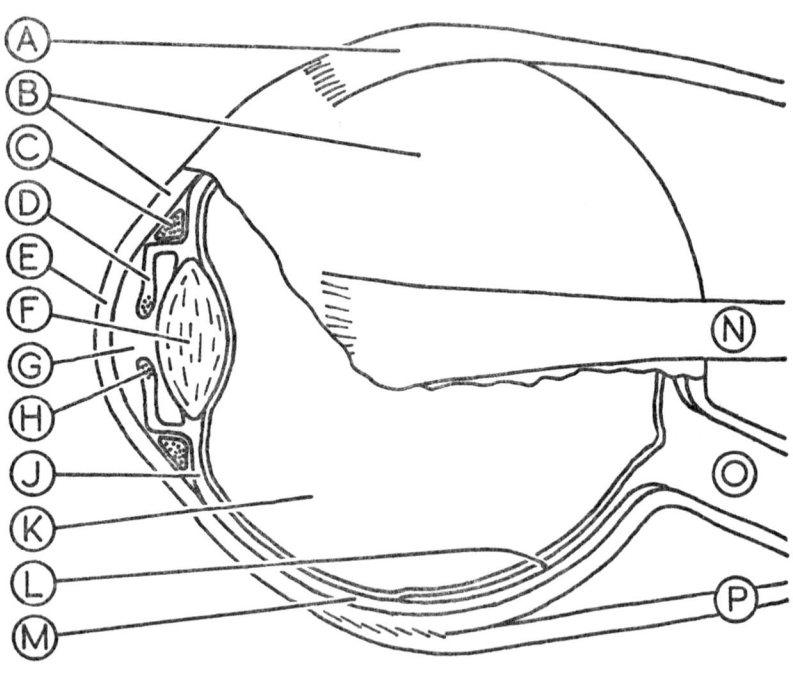

FIG. 1.—*Diagrammatic presentation of the Right Eye*

(As seen from above, and partly sectioned to show internal structures)

A. *External Rectus*, one of the extrinsic muscles. When this contracts it pulls the eye outward—*i.e.*, to the side.

B. *Sclera*. The tough, white outer coat of the eyeball.

C. *Ciliary Muscle*, responsible for altering the focus of the lens. As the muscular ring contracts, the convexity (" bulge ") of the lens increases, due to pressure within the lens.

D. *Iris*. The coloured ring which regulates the entry of light into the eye.

E. *Cornea*. The domed, transparent part of the sclera, in front of the iris and lens.

F. *Lens*. Transparent and elastic, which forms images on the retina.

G. *Aqueous Humour*. A clear, nutrient fluid filling the space behind the cornea, and which bathes the lens and inner surface of the cornea.

H. *Sphincter* of the Iris, a ring of muscle which constricts the aperture (" pupil ") of the iris.

J. *Suspensory Ligament*. An elastic ring which supports the lens and keeps it under tension—*i.e.*, partly flattened—except when counteracted by the ciliary muscle.

K. *Vitreous Humour*, a clear jelly which fills the space between the lens and the retina.

L. *Retina*, consisting of sensitive cells and nerve fibres, and continuous with the optic nerve.

M. *Choroid*, a deeply pigmented lining which keeps unwanted light from entering the eye.

N. *Superior Rectus*, the muscle which swings the eyeball upward.

O. *Optic nerve*. The large trunk of nerve fibres, continuous with the retina, and passing back into the brain.

P. *Internal Rectus*, which swings the eye inwards—towards the nose.

Eye Structure

The eye proper—as shown in Fig. 1—is a spherical body, consisting of a tough, white elastic outer layer—the *sclera*—which contains and supports the other structures. The front part of this outer coat is transparent, and forms the slightly bulging *cornea*. Immediately behind this is the *iris*, a coloured ring which can dilate or contract to regulate the amount of light entering the eye. The space between the cornea and the iris is filled with a clear nutrient fluid—the *aqueous humour*. The central hole in the iris is the *pupil*, which normally looks black, and behind this is the *lens* which forms a tiny image of the outside world on the sensitive rear inner surface of the eyeball—the *retina*. The space between the lens and the retina is filled with transparent jelly—the *vitreous body*. From the innumerable sensitive cells of the retina arise thousands of fine nerve fibres, which converge and pass out through the rear of the eyeball in a large trunk—the *optic nerve*. This nerve can be considered as an extension of the brain, and indeed the eye itself has several characteristics of a part of the brain.

In some primitive animals the eye is rigidly fixed within the head, or may even be sunk in the brain. By situating the eye at the end of a " stalk," as in man and the higher animals, *movement* becomes possible and is effected by a group of *extrinsic muscles*. These are attached to the outside of the eyeball and lie between it and the bony socket. Within the eyeball, there are also muscles which control the iris and the lens, and these are the *intrinsic* muscles of the eye.

In normal functioning, the eye is directed toward the object of attention by the extrinsic muscles, and the light reflected by the object into the eye is controlled by the iris and focused sharply by the lens on the retina. In the retina, the light is absorbed by sensitive cells, which generate and send signals through the nerve fibres to the brain for interpretation. This outline, however, gives only the sketchiest account of the mechanism of vision. To give a little idea of the full complexity, let us take only three simple considerations : First, there are two eyes, and thus two sets of extrinsic muscles which must work together in strict harmony, so that both eyes are aimed at the same spot at any given instant. When the object is close at hand, the eyes must converge —" squint "—so that each is pointing directly at the object. With more distant viewing, the eyes have more parallel axes. Second, the human eye can not only distinguish between light and shade, but can also analyse the colours of objects. This means that the retina is composed of several different kinds of cell, each sensitive to light and shade or to a variety of colours. Third, since only a relatively small area of the retina is able to discern fine detail, the eye must be actively yet precisely moved about, so that various parts of the object are in turn focused on this sensitive area. Meantime the brain receives a rapid succession of complex messages, and almost instantaneously deduces information from these about the shape, size, colour, distance, direction, and speed of movement of the object. Occasionally, under difficult circumstances, the brain responds sluggishly, or is confused as to whether it is the external object or the eye itself which is moving. The peculiar sensations which result are not confined to alcoholics— a total abstainer, if sleepy enough, may experience the milder forms !

Factors in Perception

Normally, the brain's responses are rapid and accurate, but the rapidity and accuracy depend upon several variables. The sharper and, within limits, the brighter the image on the retina, the clearer the signals conveyed to the brain. The more precise the movements of the eye, the more effectively is the picture built up in the mind. The more fresh and alert the brain cells, the quicker the response—*perception*.

The brightness of the image is primarily dependent upon external conditions, but the other factors are all determined essentially by the general fitness of the individual. When the entire visual mechanism is healthy and well-nourished, sight is normal. When, in any part, the response is dulled by malnutrition or low vitality, the vision is defective.

The memory centres play a particularly vital part in the mechanism of vision, since they make possible recognition and association.

In all functionings of the brain and sense organs, familiar objects, sensations and situations are more quickly and easily identified than are unusual or new experiences. In some instances this is patently obvious, but the importance of recognition as it applies to eyesight is not always appreciated. We have all had experience of the value of " knowing what to look for " in the broader sense. Quite literally, however, it is an essential for efficient vision. Think, for example, of how much more quickly one can read print of a familiar pattern than when it is in an unusual form. To most of us, accustomed to Roman lettering, Gothic text is almost illegible, while the reverse is true of a German brought up with the traditional lettering of his country. Even more striking, however, is the behaviour of the eye when presented with a totally new picture. My own realisation of this came most forcibly when as a student I tried to see all the tiny structures in plants and animals which the text-books assured me were there. Occasionally some item would elude me completely, and it was not until a demonstrator pointed it out that it became visible. That was quite in order : but the astonishing thing was how the particular object became from that moment strikingly obvious. Even a quick glance at a specimen after that was enough to let me see the details required. So far as that particular item was concerned, my visual mechanism was now able to function vastly more efficiently. It knew what to expect, and it had immediate reference to a previous experience. In simple language, I had become more familiar with my subject. Without an efficient system of memory and recognition, the eyesight is seriously impaired, no matter how efficient its mechanical and optical components.

CHAPTER II

MUSCLES, FOCUSING AND EXERCISE

LET us look now at a few of the more common abnormalities which may develop in conditions of excessive strain or poor health. In their crudest form, defects in the extrinsic muscles and their controls make it difficult or impossible for the eye to be accurately aimed, or the co-ordination of the two eyes may become unreliable. In a mild form the person may occasionally see a double image, due to the failure of the two eyes to merge their images properly, a condition termed *diplopia*.

In more serious cases the disorder is quite evident to the onlooker. In *nystagmus* the eyeballs are not smoothly directed towards the object, but flutter back and forth several times before settling. In very severe conditions, which may develop after prolonged strain—emotional, occupational, nutritional etc.—there may be no " settling," but a continual fluttering. In *strabismus* —squint—the two eyes do not point in the same direction. Strabismus may be *internal* or *external*, depending upon whether the axes of the eyes converge or diverge. Nystagmus and strabismus are most often due directly to nervous strains, which in turn may be caused by a variety of circumstances. Although it is perhaps of minor practical importance, it is interesting that an abnormal air-pressure on the outside of the eardrum can produce an immediate nystagmus in some people. More significant are the commoner predisposing causes which include : an over-sensitive nature, often coupled with introspection ; dietary errors involving excess sugars and starches ; intake of drugs such as tea, coffee, tobacco or alcohol ; poor posture, especially involving the neck ; and a poor heredity—*i.e.*, the parents have made mistakes of a similar nature.

Nervous Imbalance

Squint is frequently the outward sign of a distress which, occurring in another individual, might lead to such manifestations as left-handedness, stammering or asthma. Obviously, any attempt to correct such a condition by treating the eyes alone is bound to fail. Optical or mechanical correction may, of course, be effected, but if the basic mental conflict remains there will be an inevitable tendency to recurrence. Alternatively, in some cases, there may be a breakdown of some other part as evidence of distress. No matter how much the specialist may prefer to believe otherwise, to " cure " (suppress) one symptom only to have another appear, is not a satisfactory solution. In fact it does not cure anything. To produce a genuine cure it is essential to remove both the primary cause and any residual stresses. In a long-standing case, bad habits, both in thought and muscular control, may continue even when the original strain has been completely removed. Marked success has attended treatment consisting of improvement in the general nutrition, followed by a course of deliberate re-education to give back the eyes their confidence. Such simple devices as a cover on the " good " or dominant eye, to compel the other to function, can be rapidly effective once nutrition is restored to normal, and the tensions have been eased. But the same treatment applied without preliminary or simultaneous attention to the general physical and emotional background may quite easily produce even greater distress in the vision, or further breakdown elsewhere in the body.

The primary causes of nystagmus may be very similar to those of squint, but whereas the emotional aspect is usually dominant in squint, in nystagmus it is more common for physical strains to play the larger part. Low vitality or difficult working conditions—typically very dim lighting—add to the emotional difficulties, and produce a localised hysteria in the muscles. In the early stages, the nervous controls exhibit delayed action, and their signals lack precision. The result is a simple " looseness " or backlash in the eye movements. Building up a reserve of vitality and improving the external physical conditions may be more immediately important than local exercises or any form of psychological treatment.

The extrinsic muscles may malfunction in many other ways. It is possible for one or more muscles to be over-stimulated, or to be constantly exerting themselves against each other—excessive tone. For instance, the muscle which swings the eye inward (towards the nose) may exert too strong a pull. To compensate, and so keep the eye in its normal forward position, the opposing muscle has to exert an equivalent tension. This tug-of-war distorts the elastic eyeball, and the image on the retina is affected. This is one cause of *astigmatism*, a condition in which, for example, horizontal lines are seen sharply, but vertical lines appear fuzzy. Such muscular imbalance is closely connected with general nervous distress, and is usually more evident in worry or excitement. The excess muscular tension, apart from causing a direct disturbance of vision, will in time result in fatigue and aching of the muscles.

Comfort Not Enough

Reflecting the general condition of the body, the muscles of the eye may all be in a state of too little or excess tone—they may be flabby or highly strung. Flabbiness produces no particular discomfort, but is evidenced by sluggish and inaccurate control. Excess tensions, however, may not only give rise to acute discomfort, but may in time alter the natural shape of the eyeball. If this occurs, the individual may find difficulty in seeing sharply either at a distance or close at hand. If non-uniform distortions occur, the vision may be indistinct—astigmatic—at all distances.

This brings us to the mechanism of focusing—a point around which there has been much controversy. Some years ago Dr W. H. Bates of New York claimed that the generally accepted theory was false. Instead of being carried out by alteration in the shape of the lens, as is usually believed, Dr. Bates was satisfied that focusing was effected by a lengthening or shortening of the eyeball produced by pressures of the extrinsic muscles. On the basis of this theory, Dr. Bates produced his now famous system of treatment, which consists largely of exercises for these muscles. His treatment was successful, and he gained a considerable following, particularly among unorthodox practitioners. His original book—*Perfect Sight Without Glasses*—set the fashion for quite a number of similar publications. Almost without exception, his followers have accepted his theory of the focusing mechanism.

The Art of Seeing

A notable exception is Aldous Huxley. In *The Art of Seeing* he virtually suggests that the Bates theory is untenable, but emphasises that this point is of little practical consequence : the essential fact being the effectiveness of the treatment. A considerable time before Huxley's writing, however, several Nature Cure practitioners in this country had come to a similar conclusion. They freely recommended many of Bates' exercises, although making it clear that they did not subscribe to all his theories.

The examples which Bates and his followers have brought forward as proofs have so far only shown that his claim is justified in certain—abnormal—cases. They do not show that it is generally true or that it applies to normally healthy people. To be more specific : Bates found (1) that in some cases the lens did not alter its shape in focusing ; (2) that in others where the lens had been surgically removed, focusing was still possible. From these, and similar observations, he deduced as the only possible explanation that the shape of the eyeball must be deliberately changed by the extrinsic muscles. (See Fig. 1 : p. 14.)

So far as it applies to exceptional cases—such as non-elastic or absent lens—his reasoning was sound. It is readily demonstrable that the shape of the eyeball can be altered by muscular or other external pressures ; also that the expected alterations in focus result as the distance of the lens from the retina is changed. For example, a short-sighted person can temporarily improve his distant sight by exerting a firm pressure for a few moments on the front of his eyeballs. The pressure shortens these and so gives—for a while—sharper vision of distant objects. (Note well, this is an experiment—not a treatment !) It does not matter whether the short-sightedness is due to abnormality of the lens or of the eyeball. The optical arrangement of the eye is basically the same as that of a camera and, as most photographers know, there are two ways in which the focus of a camera can be adjusted. The distance of the lens from the film may be varied, or the structure of the lens itself may be altered. These methods are not mutually exclusive, but with any given camera one will be normal. In some animals the eyeball does lengthen and shorten to alter focus, but there can be little doubt that in normal human eyesight it is alteration in the shape of the lens which provides focusing for far and near objects. Alteration of the shape of the eyeball is the *emergency* method.[1]

A number of simple confirmations of this—both practical and philosophical—are available, but need not concern us now. It is enough to observe that the shape of a normal eyeball is practically constant, and the focusing is carried out by the action of a ring of ciliary muscle surrounding the lens—that is, by muscles *within* the eyeball. But in the abnormal eye, this simple and efficient device may be unable to produce clear and precise focusing, since the eyeball may be distorted and the lens may be inelastic and deformed. The ball may be distorted by pressure of the external muscles, by weakness in its own structure, or by pressure of the fluids it contains. It may be elongated or flattened in any direction.

---

[1] Just as a man who has lost his vocal chords can sometimes be trained to " speak " by swallowing air and regurgitating it through an artificial larynx, so can focusing sometimes be effected by the extrinsic muscles—but in neither case should the function be considered " normal."

Lens Defects

The lens may be too bulgy, too flat, or uneven : the muscular and elastic fibres which control it may be flabby, tense, or unbalanced in their action. It is worth noting that every type of visual disturbance which can be caused by a distorted eyeball can also be produced by a distorted lens. This point will be discussed in detail later.

No matter what defect may be present, the controls of the body will seek to maintain sharpness of vision. Thus, for instance, if the eyeball is elongated and if for any reason its shape cannot be restored, the lens will tend to be held flatter than normal. In another case, if the lens loses its mobility, or if its elasticity is restricted, the brain may use the external muscles of the eyeball in an attempt to provide a compensating change in the shape of the ball.

Short-sightedness—*myopia*—may be due to an elongated eyeball, or to a too-convex (bulging) lens. In either case, the orthodox remedy is to place in front of the eye a concave glass (or plastic) lens, which neutralises the error and allows a sharp image to be formed on the retina. As most Nature Cure adherents will deduce, the probable effect of such an action is that the body will discontinue any effort it may have been making to compensate or to restore the parts to normal. For this reason, a common result of wearing spectacles is progressive degeneration of the eyesight. Orthodox eye-specialists admit that this seems to occur, but try to explain it away on the grounds that once his vision has been improved by the spectacles, the subject becomes more aware of his deficiencies. Having once seen clearly, the patient begins to realise how bad his natural sight is.

This is a reasonable and ingenious argument, but it does not meet the great majority of cases, in which a gradual but progressive increase in the " power " of the lenses is called for, as year follows year.

Long-sightedness—*hypermetropia*—is most commonly due to a shortened eyeball, although in elderly folk a hardened and too-flat lens can also be responsible (*presbyopia*). (See page 42.) The physical and mental background of a short-sighted individual is usually quite different from that of a far-sighted person. Relationship between physical and mental activities is often very clearly observed in our work, and eye disorders are no exception. The person with short sight is inclined to be interested in nearby things, and physical nearness is readily translated into matters of time. It is not accidental that " far-seeing " and " short-sighted " are terms with very broad meanings.

The Nervous Aspect

In any individual case it may not be easy to determine whether the defective eyesight is a primary cause of restricted mental outlook, or whether the rôles are reversed. The third possibility—that the mental and visual abnormalities are both due to other factors—is just as likely to be true. Lest the long-sighted person should feel too superior, it is worth noting that much of the world's unhappiness has been brought about by men who took too long and broad a view, and ignored the finer details nearer home ! " The eyes of the fool are on the ends of the earth." Healthy eyesight, like healthy thinking, should be balanced.

This gives a clue to part of the treatment of short and long-sightedness : the restoration of general nervous balance. With this muscular tone becomes normal—

strains ease, and flabbiness is taken up. The nourishment and oxygenation of the defective parts must be improved. Dietetic and manipulative attention may be essential. But above all, and just as with any lazy or inefficient part of the body, the attention of the system must be drawn to the condition and free circulation of blood encouraged.

These two last can be effected and direct benefit obtained by exercises for the muscles involved. A normal, healthy muscle only remains so if it is frequently in action and regularly used to its full range of movement. Any muscle which is used over only a small part of its range is liable to lose the ability to move fully. Spectacles are particularly harmful in this respect, since, instead of following, or looking for, an object with the eyes only, the tendency is for the whole head to be moved. The eyeball thus becomes relatively immobile, and its muscles and circulation suffer from inactivity. (The head-movements, however, may keep the neck-muscles in good tone, so encouraging a freer circulation to the head, including the brain. This may in some degree compensate for the loss of natural exercise.)

The Importance of Movement . . .

Since lack of full movement seriously affects a muscle, it is important to try to avoid small, repeated, tense eye actions as much as possible, and to perform full, easy movements fairly frequently. In reading, for instance, it is usual for the page to be held at a fixed position, while the movements of the eye are small, and uniform. Just as an arm aches if it is held for long in one position, so the intrinsic eye muscles tend to become exhausted and irritated.

It is easy to avoid strain of this kind. For example, if one lifts the eyes every few lines, and looks at some distant object for a second or two, the muscles will remain comfortable for quite long spells. Again, the book, or the head, can be gently moved, so that the distance between eye and page is frequently altered. If much reading has to be done, another way of providing the muscles with a change of occupation is to hold the page at an angle, so that instead of simply swinging from side to side, the eye travels diagonally.

The muscles of the eye are quite easily exercised, although because of their invisibility it is necessary to know something of their actions and effects when selecting exercises for them. As already mentioned, most of Bates' original exercises are excellent. They have been described in many writings.

Bates' own book is published in this country by Faber, under the title *Good Sight Without Glasses*, and Aldous Huxley's *The Art of Seeing* is published by Chatto and Windus. Huxley, in addition to describing the Bates' exercises, discusses at length the mental processes of seeing—a valuable complement to the more physical considerations. (Huxley's book, which expresses much of the Nature Cure philosophy, was strongly resented by the orthodox profession when it appeared. The Southport Libraries Committee, for instance, banned it on the advice of local medicos.)

Two main groups of muscles should be exercised : the extrinsic muscles, which move the eyeball, and the intrinsic muscles, which control the iris and the lens. In addition, it is helpful to use muscles related to the eyesocket, such as those of the eyelids and face, so that the local circulation and nervous tone may be improved.

. . . and Rest

All muscles welcome a brief rest. Movement is preferred to fixed tension, but occasional relaxation is also important. To rest the muscles of the eye, Bates' technique of " palming " is helpful. In this, the eyes are covered with the slightly cupped palms of the hands— the fingers crossing on the forehead. The elbows should rest on the lap, or on a table, and the head is inclined forward. The palms keep out the light, so allowing the controls to relax. (Relaxation does not occur so completely when the lids are closed in the attempt to exclude light.) The eyes are kept covered for at least half a minute, or often very much longer, during which time there ought to be a feeling of general relaxation and comfort. There should be a gradual fading out of any visual pattern and blotches, which are usually evident when the eyes are first covered. It is important that the palms should exert no pressure on the eyeballs, and the weight of the head should be taken on the hands so that the neck muscles are relaxed.

For active exercise, a simple routine should be followed to ensure that each muscle is given due attention. There are two basic requirements in mind : the eyes should be moved in *every* direction as far as they will go, and they should be called upon to focus on both very near and distant objects. Normally, it is best to begin each set of exercises with simple movements, gradually increasing the complexity and speed.

An easy first movement is to swing the eyes from one side to the other, quite slowly and deliberately, and then back again. The movement should be taken to the comfortable limit in each direction, and after a few repetitions the eyes can be coaxed to move just a little further round than is comfortable. So long as the swing is slow and steady, there is no danger whatever in the slight feeling of strain, although enthusiasm must be tempered with common sense. Jerky movements should be avoided, and actual pain should not occur.

This movement may be repeated a dozen times or more. The number of repetitions for any exercise is variable, and depends on the state of the individual. If any movement becomes irritating or painful, it should be discontinued immediately, although not forgotten at the next session of exercise.

Next, swing the eyes upward and downward in similar fashion to the first movement.

The following is slightly more complex : instead of swinging the eyes horizontally from one side to the other, let the glance loop upward, as though following a rainbow from end to end. Then make the same movement with a downward swing.

After several repetitions of each, try making complete circles, in each direction, until the movement becomes easy and smooth.

To give the controls a more interesting task, start by looking straight ahead, and then slowly roll the eyes as though following an outward spiral, so that after about three revolutions the eye is following the widest possible circle. Make a few revolutions of this circle, and then start again at the centre, but this time revolve in the opposite direction.

The extrinsic muscles have by these movements been tensed and relaxed to their limits, in a slow and deliberate fashion. Also, the co-ordination has been exercised and tested. If any particular movement seems

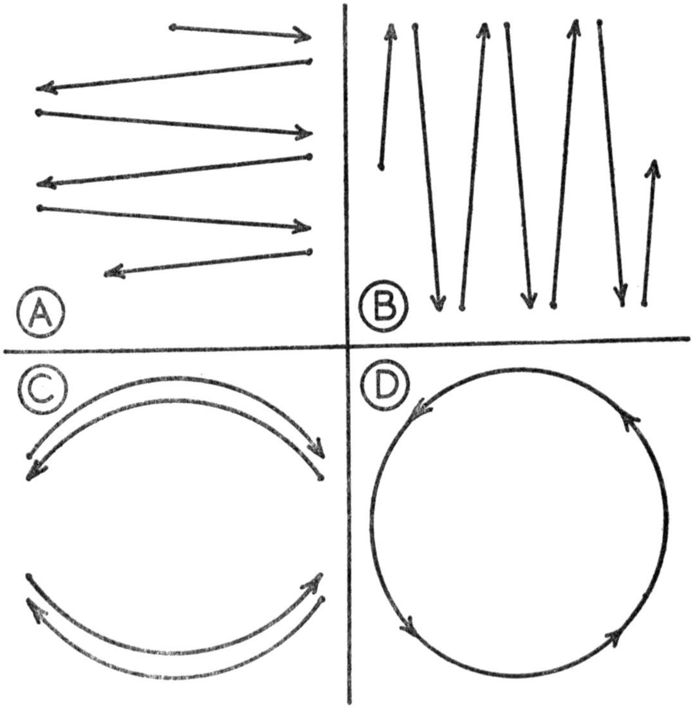

FIG. 2.—*Eye Exercises in Diagram Form.*

A. Swinging from side to side.
B. Swinging up and down.
C. Looping upward and downward from side **to side.**
D. Circling in both directions.

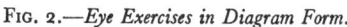

FIG. 2.—*Eye Exercises in Diagram Form.*

E. Spiralling outward in both directions.

F. Darting outward in all directions.

G. Focusing near and far.

H. Focusing on objects of varying distance and
    brightness.

difficult, that is the one to which the greatest attention should be given.

Imagination

The next stage is to perform the same movements as already described, but more rapidly. In this case, the purpose is mainly to encourage circulation in the muscles by vigorous activity, and accordingly—in the early stages at least—the movements may not be so precise as when performed slowly.

To help in making rapid, full movements, try making mental pictures of occupations such as watching a very fast game of tennis, as seen from one end of the net !

As the final exercise of this group, look straight ahead and then let the eyes dart outward rapidly, as though looking in turn at each figure on a large, close clock-face, returning to the centre between each outward sweep.

Convergence

The next group of exercises involves the mechanism of accommodation, of which one important function is the convergence of the two eyes when looking at nearby objects.

Starting with a simple exercise, as usual, hold up a finger about six inches in front of the nose, and look quite deliberately at the tip of the finger, and then just as deliberately at something far off—that is, at least twenty feet away. Some folk may find six inches uncomfortably close, while others, particularly youngsters, will find that they can easily see a finger almost touching the nose. Repeat the movement slowly about a dozen times, and then try carrying it out as rapidly as possible, another dozen times.

So far we have not given our immediate attention

to focusing, although the last-mentioned exercise can be valuable for the focusing mechanism. Most people find that although it is possible to make the " two fingers become one " quite rapidly when returning from distant sight, there may be quite a detectable pause before the detail of the finger-tip comes into sharp focus. With many, and particularly the older folk, the finger may not come into sharp focus at all. These people should extend the arm slowly until the finger becomes sharp. (This will occur at a shorter distance in bright light than in dim lighting.)

The exercise should then be repeated, with particular care that the finger is seen sharply before looking off into the distance, and similarly with the distant object before returning. Many people will be surprised how long it takes their eyes to adjust themselves precisely in a severe test of this kind. With a little practice, however, the speed and accuracy should improve considerably.

When this exercise has been mastered, it can be made one degree more intensive by selecting—say—four objects at different distances and in different directions, and looking at each in rapid succession. Typical positions would be : nine inches away and to the right ; two feet, and to the left ; six feet, upward ; and far off, straight ahead. (The first could be a finger, the second a book, the third part of a window-frame, and the last a church spire, as in Fig. 2.) There is no need whatever to make elaborate preparations, and such an exercise can be performed quite unobtrusively at any time and in almost any surroundings. This exercise, incidentally, directly affects the iris control. On changing attention from an indoor to an outdoor object, in addition to altering their position, convergence and focusing, the eyes are also called upon to close the iris apertures so that the retina is not dazzled by the brighter lighting. The iris control can be stimulated by any marked change in the illumination. (In passing, it should be mentioned that the iris cannot respond to very rapid alternations of light and dark. With slow flicker-ings—say three or four per second—there is a very marked irritation of the control centres, which seem to be just on the point of " ordering " an alteration in the iris when the light changes back, and the message has to be stopped—just in time for another change to set off another message. Although the effect is liable to vary with each individual, white light interrupted several times per second usually gives the impression of *coloured* flashes. If the interruptions are made slightly more rapid, the eye sees a grey flickering, while if the inter-ruptions occur more than about fifty times per second, the impression is of steady illumination. This makes possible the cinematograph, TV and the use of fluores-cent lighting. With both the picture screen and the fluorescent tube, however, flicker is quite evident if the light is observed out of the *side* of the eye, when either the eye or any object is moved. The central area of the retina is less sensitive to changes in brightness than the outer parts, as well as having other peculiarities as discussed on page 49.)

To encourage the response of the iris, alternating one's glance between a dark corner and a bright window is sufficient, although a more intense stimulus is provided by " sunning " (p. 47). A simple method of exercising most of the eye muscles and controls simultaneously is to stand with the face about six inches from a door-post, or any other clearly defined vertical strip, and run the attention rapidly up and down an edge. After several repetitions, a similar exercise may be performed with a horizontal line such as a bookshelf. The head, of course, may be turned into various positions so that a single guide line serves for all movements. After the vertical and horizontal movements, try diagonals—top left to bottom right, and top right to bottom left.

A Water Treatment

There is no reason why eye exercises should not be combined with other therapeutic activities. An effective morning and evening application consists of plunging the face into a basin of cold water, opening the eyes, and looking up, down, left and right. A second set of movements can then be performed in the diagonal directions.

The same eye movements can be carried out " dry," combined with neck movements. For this a mirror helps. Face the mirror, and look at your own eyes. Then keeping your attention fixed, move the head in all directions—back and forward, side to side, turning and rolling. This effectively assists the circulation to the head, and so gives a dual benefit.

As an impromptu exercise to increase the general efficiency and alertness of the eye's mechanisms, it is helpful to practise trying to see objects sharply and distinctly with a single quick glance. The objects should be at all distances, and in light ranging from full sun to indoor shadow.

(Other more general exercises which may benefit the eyesight are described in Chapter VIII.)

CHAPTER III

FOCUSING ABNORMALITIES

LET us now consider in greater detail the focusing mechanism and some of its commoner derangements. As we have already seen, the normal eyeball is practically spherical, with a slight bulge to the front—the cornea. In Fig. 3 the normal mechanism of focusing is shown in the figures A and B. In A, the "resting" position, the lens is flattened, and light rays arriving from a distant point (far to the left of the diagram) are brought to a sharp point on the retina. When a nearer object is viewed, as in B, the active or tense position is assumed : the lens is made more convex, so that again each point of the object forms a sharp point on the retina.

Note that the more convex (bulging) the lens, the more are the rays deflected—brought together—by it. The nearer the object, the greater the convexity required to produce a sharp image. For simplicity only one point of the object is shown, in the form of a star, to indicate that light from the point radiates in all directions. For focusing to be effective, all the rays entering the eye from the point must be caused to coincide in a microscopic area of the retina. In the diagram, the upper ray from the object is deflected, by the lens, down towards the centre of the retina. The lower ray is deflected upward to the same point. A ray striking the centre of the lens would pass straight through, without deviation, and coincide with the other two. Similar paths are followed by rays arriving to the right and left of the

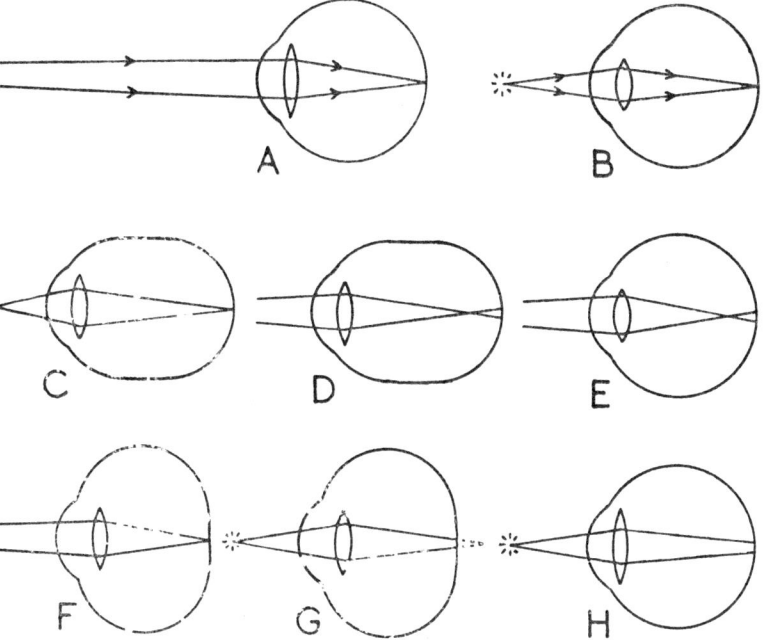

FIG. 3.—*Diagrammatic presentation of Normal and Abnormal Eyeballs and Lenses.*

A. *Normal :* Focused on distant object : lens held flat.
B. *Normal :* Focused on near object : lens distended.
C. *Elongated Eyeball :* Focuses most easily on near objects.
D. *Elongated Eyeball :* Distant Objects not easily focused.
E. *Eyeball Normal,* but Lens over-distended : distant objects not easily focused.
F. *Shortened Eyeball :* Focuses most easily on distant objects.
G. *Shortened Eyeball :* Near objects not easily focused.
H. *Eyeball Normal,* but lens flattened : near objects not easily focused.
     (Fuller explanation in text.)

lens centre, so that when focusing is exact, the rays of light form two cones, both based in the lens. The apex of one cone lies on the object, the apex of the other on the retina. The complete image is formed by a large number of such points. Although in the diagram the near object is shown as very close to the eye, in fact the shortest distance at which an object can be sharply focused, in a young adult, is about four inches. (At the other end of the scale, no alteration in focusing is required for objects between about twenty feet and infinity.)

Normally the alteration in the shape of the lens is effected so rapidly that many people are quite unaware of its action. They transfer their attention from a near object to a far distant point, and the necessary adjustment is so effortless that it is almost undetectable.

Short-sight

The second row of figures represent near-sighted eyes. C and D show short-sight (myopia) due to an elongated eyeball, which may be caused by such disorders as abnormal pressures within the eyeball, or by tensions in the extrinsic muscles. When the lens is held in its position of medium tension (as shown), the eye is focused for near objects. Far objects cannot be sharply seen, since, as shown in D, the rays are brought to a point in front of the retina, and then spread out forming a third, very small, cone before reaching its surface. In E another type of myopia is shown. In this, the eyeball is normal in shape, but the lens is excessively convex. Even when held as flat as possible the lens is so " strong " that it forms the image of a distant object " too soon "—i.e., short of the retina. The rays reach the retina over a patch instead of in a point : that is, the image is fuzzy.

The sharpness of the image can be improved by two external aids. Firstly : partial improvement will result from any narrowing of the cone of rays reaching the lens. We have already mentioned that the iris constricts its aperture (pupil) in bright light. As the iris closes, fewer diverging rays are admitted, and correspondingly the fuzziness is diminished. A bright light, then, favours sharp vision, whereas dim lighting is like to reduce acuity, at the same time producing a dull image on the retina. Even people with normal sight can usually improve the clarity of detail by a simple variation of this method, i.e., by looking through a very small aperture such as the hole made by poking the point of a pencil through a thin card. A similar effect is produced by half-closing the eyelids—hence the typical " screwed-up " grimace of the short-sighted person trying to look far off (also of the long-sighted person trying to thread a needle). The other method is, of course, the use of an auxiliary lens to neutralise the optical error. Whether the short-sightedness is due to an elongated eyeball or to an over-distended lens, distant vision will be improved by placing a concave (" hollow ") lens in front of the eye. However, both of these are artificial gains. Genuine improvement can only be effected either by restoration of the lens or eyeball to normal shape, or, where this is impossible or very difficult, by the body producing a deliberate deformation of either to compensate for the defect in the other. Thus, if the lens is obstinately over-convex, e.g., because the pressures within it are too great to be overcome by the elasticity of the suspensory ligament, the eyeball may be shortened.

This shortening may be active and temporary, as in the circumstances described by Bates, or it may be permanent. Temporary—*i.e.*, controllable—shortening is likely to occur when the lens is immobile, as it enables the person to vary the focus, within limits. Permanent shortening is probable when the lens is still mobile, but for some reason its range of movements has been altered—*i.e.*, it can be made more convex than normal but cannot be held flat enough for distant viewing. Satisfactory natural adaptation of this kind, is, of course, very much more likely to occur when the bloodstream is clean and active, and the nervous controls in healthy balance.

Long-sight

The third row of figures represents long-sighted eyes. F and G show a shortened eyeball, in which distant objects can be sharply focused (F), while with a near object (G) the cone of rays does not come to a point. The dotted lines in G show that position where the rays would focus—behind the eyeball. This shortening of the eyeball may be produced by a variety of causes, often by pressure of excess fatty or other tissues within the eyesocket, tending to push the ball forward. In older people, a more common cause of long-sightedness is insufficient convexity of the lens, as shown in H. The flattened lens may result from inadequate pressure within its substance : from weakness of the ciliary muscle, or from stiffness of the suspensory ligament. (See diagram page 14.) The orthodox remedy is the provision of a convex lens to " assist " the lens of the eye.

In long-sight, as with short-sight, either the eyeball or the tension on the lens may be modified to compensate for the deficiencies of the other. In any given circumstance the acuity of vision will be determined by the balance between the primary abnormality (produced by ill-health or external strain) and the compensatory change. Always there is a degree of tension in the situation : the abnormality is constantly " coaxed " to revert to normal, and the compensatory effect is being similarly encouraged to be " more helpful." This tension is extremely valuable, ensuring that every possible advantage is taken of improving circumstances. In this, alert nervous controls are essential for maximum efficiency.

This explains our principal objection to the use of spectacles : by neutralising tensions, they diminish self-healing and discourage adaptability in the tissues. Their very efficiency condemns them. Just as with an individual, comfortable mediocrity and absence of incentives—whether painful or pleasant—tend toward laziness and stagnation.

It must be mentioned that there are two quite common conditions in which we have no quarrel with the use of spectacles. First, in elderly folk it may be impossible to restore the focusing mechanism to full action. In most of these cases the lens has become stiff, and does not distend as required for focusing on nearby objects. For these people, reading spectacles are very helpful, since they make possible a sharp image on the retina, while allowing the muscle of the lens to remain at rest. This argument can, of course, be advanced in the case of younger folk engaged in close work of a continuous nature. Except in watchmaking, and similar exacting occupations, however, the strain of constant close focusing can be readily, and much more healthily, eased by the simple process of giving the eye-muscles frequent exercise, as suggested on page 29.

Avoid " Correction "

Reading spectacles ought to be simply " magnifying lenses," and should not be stronger than the individual finds necessary for comfort. It is most desirable that *there should be no " correction " in the lenses*, since this provision tends to perpetuate any muscular or structural imbalance. (See below.) It is important that the glasses should not *always* be worn for reading : the person should occasionally ask his eyes to do their unaided best for a minute or two. In this way any tendency to further deterioration may be minimised.

The other case occurs when the lens of the eye has been surgically removed. *Enucleation* is sometimes performed as a treatment for cataract, and although we find that it is often possible to clear slight cataract by natural methods, there is no way of restoring the function of an eye *after* operation except by the provision of an external lens. It is true, however, that very few of these mutilating operations would be undertaken if spectacles were not so readily available.

Astigmatism

Apart from the simple abnormalities already described, a very common condition occurs when the lens or eyeball is asymmetrically distorted. It is then possible for the focusing to be effective in one plane, and not in another. Thus in astigmatism one might find that the lens as seen from above is as in B of Fig. 3, while from the side it is as in H. That is, the lens is under greater tension upward and downward than from side to side. The point (represented by the star) then cannot give a point image on the retina. Instead, it will produce a vertical line. Deformity of the cornea can produce exactly similar distortion of the image.

Astigmatism due to distortion of the lens is usually very much more noticeable with distant objects than when looking at nearby things. This is probably due to the relaxed state of the ciliary muscle when the eye is focused for distance. Uneven pressures and tensions in the lens are unopposed by the ciliary muscles which, when active, are capable of balancing the strains to produce a more regularly shaped lens. Whether the abnormality is in the lens or the eyeball as a whole, exercise and improved nutrition are helpful in encouraging a return to normal.

CHAPTER IV

RETINAL DEFECTS AND DANGERS

TURNING now to the optical structures themselves, we find many possible derangements of the cornea, iris, lens and retina. Normally, the cornea and lens are highly transparent, but if the bloodstream is choked with wastes, and particularly if the blood pressure is high, there is a tendency for either of these structures to become cloudy. The lens is particularly liable to be affected, as in *cataract*, which can be seen from outside as a milky cloudiness behind the pupil. To the patient it appears as a dullness or mistiness of vision. When the pressure of the aqueous humour (page 14) is greatly excessive, a somewhat similar but acutely painful condition results, called *glaucoma*. (For other symptoms of glaucoma see page 63.) In some cases, all that is required to effect a rapid clearing of these conditions is a change in diet plus stimulation of the blood-cleansing organs by manipulative or hydropathic means. Cutting down starches and liquids drastically, and increasing the proportion of fresh vegetables are the most commonly indicated changes.[1] The blood should in time become less laden with wastes, and more nutrient, so encouraging the structures to return to their normal condition. Since high blood pressure is a frequent immediate cause of distress, the restriction of liquids, and of thirst-producing foods and condiments, is a particularly important requirement.[2]

[1] See also footnote, p. 92.
[2] For fuller instructions, see *High and Low Blood Pressure*, by James C. Thomson.

The iris should respond to changes in illumination, closing in bright sunlight, and opening in dim light. If the nervous state of the individual is abnormal, the iris may be unusually dilated or constricted. Thus a large pupil in sunlight is a sign either of very insensitive vision, or of nervous exhaustion. Both, of course, may be due to a common cause. A very small pupil in dim lighting indicates high nervous tension, and usually a toxic bloodsteam. Occasionally one encounters an iris in which the pupil is not circular, but irregular in shape. This may be the result of accidental damage, or due to congenital defect. In these cases the irregularity is unlikely to have any particular significance and is rarely amenable to treatment. Sometimes, however, the condition is due to serious lack of balance in the nervous controls, and reflects acute distress within the nervous system as a whole. It is comparable with the unbalanced state of the extrinsic muscles, already discussed, and indicates a need for improving the individual's general condition.

Exercising the Iris

To exercise the nervous reflexes and muscle fibres of the iris, a simple method is to face a bright light—such as a white cloud in the sky—and cover the eyes, as in palming, for a few seconds. Remove the hands, and allow the light to fall on the open eye for a similar interval. Cover and repeat perhaps a dozen times. A more vigorous treatment of the same type—" sunning " —can be performed by closing the lids while facing the sun, and blinking the eyes open momentarily. " Momentarily " is the operative word : do not be misled by the orthodox critics who deride the (imaginary) technique of " gazing at the sun ! "

The Blind Spot

Fig. 4 demonstrates one of the limitations of the retina. In the small area through which the optic nerve enters the eyeball, the retina is blind. The nerve fibres occupy the entire space, and there are practically no sensitive cells. Very few people realise that the image on the retina is thus incompletely recorded, unless some unusual set of circumstances occurs—such as those of the present experiment.

RIGHT **LEFT**

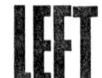

FIG. 4.—*To demonstrate the blind spot—the point where the optic nerve enters the retina, and where the retina does not respond to light—close the left eye, and at a distance of about 15 inches, fix the gaze of the right eye on the word " RIGHT." Now bring the page gradually nearer and at a certain point the word " LEFT " will vanish.*

It may be wondered why we are not continually aware of the blind spot in each retina, in the form of a dark patch on the visible image. Part of the explanation, of course, is that the normal person has two eyes, and the detail lacking from one eye's signal is supplied by the other. The total conscious impression is produced by the fusion of the two images in the brain. A more direct answer is that the sensory system is actuated by positive impulses. Where there is no sensitive cell there can be no nervous impulse, and accordingly the brain is unaware of the existence of the area concerned. (Also, if a *steady* signal does reach the brain, it tends to be progressively disregarded.)

If, for any reason, an insensitive area were suddenly to develop at some other point in the retina, the owner would most certainly be acutely aware of it—for a time. But gradually the awareness would pass as the brain adapted itself to the failure of the area. Eventually, the individual might be quite ready to believe that his vision had returned to normal, unless some unusual incident were to demonstrate otherwise. The normal person has always had the blind spot, and accordingly has no previous " perfection " to make him aware of his deficiency. The young child very quickly learns to move the eyes about so that the image which at one instant falls on a blind spot is rapidly moved to a sensitive area. The brain learns to store and correlate the impressions so that a complete picture is presented to the consciousness. This in part explains why so many drugs have an effect on the sight. Anything which weakens the memory or reduces the reasoning powers interferes with vital links in the visual chain. Conversely, an alert mind is essential to efficient vision.

The Retina

The structure of the retina is peculiar in other ways. The sensitivity varies over its surface, so that we find the centre of the retina less sensitive to dim lights than the surrounding area. On a dark night one can detect vague shapes out of the sides of the eye, but when one tries to see a shape more clearly, by looking straight at it, the images fade out. By looking straight at an object one brings its image over the area of sharpest vision, but there must be relatively good illumination of the object before the cells in this area are affected.

The fact that only a small area of the retina can distinguish fine details is not often realised by the layman. In normal eyesight, the vision appears to be full of detail, over a wide area. This is due to the ability of the eye to shift its attention rapidly from point to point, and of the brain to co-ordinate the successive messages into a comprehensible whole. The ability of the retina to distinguish different colours also varies over its surface, and is very much reduced in dim light. The brighter the illumination, the more clearly are colours distinguished. Think of how the grey surroundings of a dull, rainy day become brilliant mosaics under summer sunshine.

The retina can be damaged or deranged in a number of ways. For efficient functioning, the cells of the retina must be continually cleansed and adequately supplied with replenishing materials. The substance which is affected by light, and which generates the nervous signal—visual purple—is readily produced by the healthy body. If the diet is deficient in fresh foods, particularly green and root vegetables, the retina becomes impoverished and unable to generate strong signals. Just as in any other bodily tissue, poor circulation soon reduces the efficiency of the retina, due to fatigue. Fatigue is noticeable, even in a normal eye, when one passes from full sunshine to a dark room. For the first few seconds little can be seen, but fairly rapidly the sensitivity of the retina is restored, and one is able to distinguish details, even in the dark corners. In a person whose health is poor, fatigue is very much more noticeable. It may take many minutes for the eye to regain satisfactory vision.

Night Blindness

In some people the sensitivity of the retina is below normal—the person may be " night-blind " and cannot see at all in dim light. Night blindness—*nyctalopia*—may be due to a congenital deficiency in the retina. A normal retina is provided with two kinds of sensitive cells—rods and cones. The rods appear to be sensitive to light and dark only, while the cones can distinguish colours. But the cones require much brighter light to function than the rods. (Hence the increasing intensity of colours in bright light, as noted above.) Rods are almost absent from the area of sharpest vision—the *macula*—which is accordingly insensitive in very dim lights.

With an abnormal retina, the proportions and positions of these two kinds of cell may be altered. If the rods are deficient in number, the eye will still be able to see sharply and clearly in bright light, but not in dim light. If the cones are deficient, colour-sense will be poor, and the person may be dazzled in bright daylight—*photophobia*. (In a normal eye, the rods are " dazzled " in bright sunlight, but the less sensitive cones still produce satisfactory vision.)

However, such deficiencies need not necessarily be congenital, or even permanent. Very often they are mere symptoms of ill-health, and in such cases they usually respond quite rapidly to a general improvement in health, especially when encouraged by attention to the circulation in the head and dietetic requirements. The retina is an extremely active element in the visual process, and accordingly it is very rapidly affected by changes in the bloodstream. All the time the individual sees anything, the active substance of the sensitive cells is being consumed. To maintain supplies and ensure satisfactory cleansing, not only must the diet be adequate in the essential raw materials, but the digestive organs must be in good order, respiration must be effective, and the circulation must be free and vigorous.

Abdominal exercises and deep breathing may be just as essential parts of the treatment as the more obvious attentions to diet, neck exercises and the eyes themselves.

Invisible Dangers

There is one other important point which concerns the retina. Its tissues may be injured, or even permanently damaged by " light " which is not detected by the eye. The eye can respond to only a very small section of the wide range of radiant energies. (The general terms " electro-magnetic vibrations " or " ether waves " are commonly used to describe a vast scale, which extends from the relatively slow vibrations emitted by a long-wave radio station to the almost inconceivably rapid oscillations of cosmic rays. Visible light occurs somewhere about the middle of the scale.)

The human eye can detect and distinguish different kinds of light, from deep red at one end of the spectrum to violet at the other. (The red rays have a lower rate of vibration than the violet : with orange, yellow, green and blue intermediate.) But most forms of illuminant emit appreciable amounts of radiation outside the visible range. Those rays which have a slightly slower rate of vibration than visible reds are called " infra-red," while those beyond the violet are called " ultra-violet."

Infra-red radiation is quite readily detectable by the skin, as a sensation of warmth. Ultra-violet, however, cannot be immediately detected by the human body. (Some insects are sensitive to light which is beyond the violet of human vision.) The delayed effects of ultra-violet on the skin, however, are often quite noticeable, as in the case of acute sunburn : but there the awareness comes too late ! Both ultra-violet and infra-red " light " enter the human eye, to be focused on the retina by the lens, although not quite as sharply as visible rays. In most circumstances, the radiation from any intense source contains sufficient visible light to warn the mechanisms of the eye to take protective action. But not always. Artificial sun lamps, for instance, and particularly the mercury vapour type, emit ultra-violet light out of all proportion to the visible. Accordingly it is customary for the user to wear dense protective goggles, which keep out the ultra-violet, while allowing just enough visible light to pass that the person can see what is going on.

Sun Glasses

Under more natural conditions excessive amounts of ultra-violet light are only encountered on these islands when the person is surrounded by highly reflective surfaces, and in unusually brilliant sunshine. Typically, this situation arises at the seaside, in high mountains, or amid snow. Less natural, but quite a common circumstance, is long-distance motor-driving. If the sun is shining brilliantly, glare from the road and other surroundings may contain enough ultra-violet to produce pain in the eyes after an hour or two. Not that every pain arising in these circumstances has a serious mean-ing. Most eye-discomfort while motoring is due solely to the constant tensions and oscillations in the muscles of the eye. Commonly these are aggravated by restricted circulation due to anxiety tensions on the neck.

Where the sunshine is really strong, however, and

is strongly reflected, it is desirable, and may be imperative, to protect the eyes by wearing dark glasses. These have the double effect of allowing the iris to relax and of absorbing a high proportion of the ultra-violet. It is quite true that a yellow glass is most likely to absorb the ultra-violet efficiently, but a coloured glass not only upsets the appearance of the world, it also produces an after-effect of disturbed colour vision, which may last for a considerable time. Crookes glass is designed to give good absorption of ultra-violet (and infra-red) while producing a relatively small reduction of visible light and without upsetting the colour balance. Incidentally, many people are under the misapprehension that if they buy sun-specs. fitted with " Crookes lenses " they are getting the best optical quality. They may be, but not necessarily so. Crookes glass can be formed into just as low-grade lenses as any other glass. Lowgrade means that the lenses, instead of being neutral, are optically distorted in some way. This defect is particularly prevalent in curved lenses. First-class sun-glasses—which are quite expensive—should have lenses which are either " optical flats " or " planominiscus " (curved).

What to Avoid

Before buying inexpensive sun-specs., a simple and effective test for optical quality is to hold them at arm's length, and look through them at some distant object, while moving the specs. about. If the glasses are good, the distant object should neither appear magnified nor diminished, and it should not " ripple " violently as the glasses are moved. With all except optically ground glasses there will be a very slight wavering. This is quite permissible for occasional use. Sun-spec. lenses made from plastics of various kinds may be effective in stopping ultra-violet, or they may not. There is no readily available way of checking this particular value in any given case, but the maker's or dealer's reputation may be some guide. Unfortunately, for every person who uses sun-specs. from necessity, there are hundreds who use them only for adornment, and accordingly there is a ready market for rubbish which may be optically dangerous. If one buys specs. with grey glass lenses, and checks them for optical quality, as suggested above, one can at least be sure that they will do no harm, and that some of the ultra-violet light will be kept out of the eyes !

Infra-Red Rays

Injury to the eye by infra-red (radiant heat) is much less common in the ordinary way, although those who handle red-hot or molten metals are liable to be affected, unless reasonable care is taken. To the novice, the intense heat is sufficient warning, but the old hand develops in his skin a resistance to heat which the eye structure cannot possibly attain. Since the cornea and lens of the eye absorb a considerable proportion of the radiant heat, they are accordingly more often injured than the retina. In extreme cases the transparent tissues of the eye become whitened, like the albumen of an egg when cooked.

Although, for most folk, the risk of gross infra-red injury to the eye is not serious, one occasionally finds cases of " mysterious " pain and fatigue due to this cause. Probably the commonest situation is that where the person sits reading or working in one position, with a coal or gas fire or an electric radiator somewhere in front of him. (Perhaps you, dear reader, at this moment ?)

The total amount of infra-red reaching the eye may be small, but because of the restricted movement of the eyeball, the image of the red-hot source is more or less constantly focused on one small area of the retina. In exactly the same way that a burning-glass placed in the sun's rays can quickly scorch the hand, so the lens of the eye can burn by concentrating the heat on a small area of the retina. Dim lighting, in which the iris is fully dilated, is the commonest circumstance in which this kind of injury occurs.

In all but the most abnormal conditions, pain or acute discomfort gives ample warning before any permanent damage is done to the eye, but temporary injury may easily occur. Then, as in all bodily conditions where repair is necessary, a rich, clean, well-aerated and free-flowing bloodstream induces more rapid and complete recovery. This applies whether the temporary blindness is acute, as, for example, where due to accidental exposure to an electric arc, or the more simple form due to entering a dark room from bright sunshine.

CHAPTER V

VISUAL DISTURBANCES

Toxic Spots

A COMMON temporary visual defect is caused by toxins in the blood reaching and interfering with the sensitive retinal cells. Coloured or dark " spots before the eyes " are accounted for by such poisons irritating or benumbing the receptor cells or their related nerve fibres. An extreme example is seen in poisoning by methyl alcohol, which appears to have a strong affinity for the optic nerve. Consumption of less than one ounce of wood spirits can produce permanent destruction of the optic nerves. The much milder " spots " are fortunately quite amenable to treatment, and can be banished by improving the activity of the major blood-cleansing organs—liver and kidneys particularly.

" Floating specks " are often confused with the above condition, but arise from a different cause. With these, there is actual obstruction in the line of vision, either on the surface of the cornea, or in the transparent structures of the eye. Dust particles may adhere quite firmly to the cornea if the flow of cleansing fluid from the tear glands is inadequate, or if blinking does not occur with sufficient frequency. Blinking should naturally occur every few seconds, but unfortunately some occupations (and disease conditions) encourage a fixed stare. Such an individual should make a deliberate effort to increase his rate of blinking, which will also stimulate the local circulation, and thereby increase the tear-gland secretion. Another exercise to the same end is tight closing of the eyes, repeated several times. (With many people this is accompanied by a rushing sound in the ears.) Almost immediately, one feels a warmth around the eyes, indicating the freer flow of blood.

On the question of blinking, the daily Press has reported Professor Lawson, of Sheffield, as finding that people who blink rapidly (frequently ?) (1) never reach high proficiency in games, (2) are the most dangerous drivers, and (3) make bad scientists. He pointed out that the more frequent the blink, the greater the proportion of time during which the eye is out of action. It may be, however, that the Professor over-simplified his case (or the exigencies of space may have caused over-compression). There is, of course, a happy medium in the frequency of blinking. A very infrequent blink —say only once or twice per minute, or less—will inevitably make for inefficient eye-cleansing. A blink every five seconds or so may be enough under clean air conditions, but in dusty, smoky or fume-laden atmospheres, even once per second may not be too often. But at these higher rates, the actual *duration* of the blink becomes important. A slow—half-second—blink would mean that the eye was in action only half the time. A blink of this duration is, however, not typical of a healthy person, whose " flicker " should be much shorter than the third-of-a-second blink which is quoted by Professor Lawson as average. A slow blink denotes relaxed nervous controls, and in all probability watery tissues, so that the lids themselves are over-weight, and the muscles acting upon them weak and sluggish. The lack of clear observation, and the tendency to lose sight of a quickly-moving ball, are more likely to be another sign of the body's encumbered and devitalised state than a direct result of the blink. It is not easy to measure accurately, but from observation I should estimate that the blink of a healthy person in an alert state only interrupts the sight for about one-tenth of a second. In the same alert state, the blink is suspended entirely while any vital action is being observed, and waits until a momentary " lull " occurs. *E.g.*, the eye remains open while the tennis-ball is in flight towards the player, but blinks during its return.

Accordingly I would incline to believe that what the Professor noted is that unhealthy people are hesitant, have poor co-ordination of muscular movements, are not alert observers, and blink sluggishly.

Floating specks can also be caused by particles of opaque tissue in the vitreous humour (the jelly-like mass occupying most of the interior of the eyeball). It is most unusual for such specks to appear suddenly, although something may cause one or more to be moved closer to the line of most acute vision, and so be noticed by the person. Most commonly, these particles are residual structures which for some reason have not been normally absorbed after the vitreous humour was formed. In some folk the particles are larger and more opaque than in others, and accordingly are more liable to cause occasional interference with vision.

There is no need for the individual to be in any way concerned about such specks, although after prolonged unhygienic living there is a distinct possibility that very noticeable specks may arise indirectly from impurities in the bloodstream. We know that waste-laden blood tends to coarsen all tissues of the body, and there is no obvious reason why the vitreous humour should be an exception.

A speck due to dust on the cornea " runs away " from one's attention, for the simple reason that in trying to look directly at it, the eyeball turns and carries the speck farther to one side. Specks in the vitreous humour are not quite so predictable. Their movement does not so rigidly follow the movement of the eye : hence their presence is usually more noticeable when the eyeball is moved rapidly.

" Flying Saucers "

Related to such specks is another phenomenon which occasionally worries those who notice it for the first time. If the eye is allowed to gaze fixedly at some brightly lit but inanimate object, such as a summer sky or white cloud, one gradually becomes aware of a peculiar " busy-ness " : a confusion of crawling luminous specks, rather like the seething activity when one lifts the stone over an ants' nest. These specks are believed to be the actual shadows of blood cells, flowing through the very delicate vessels on the surface of the retina. Normally, the visual centres ignore these shapes, but when the iris is contracted (as in bright light), the shadows are sharper, and when there is no external movement, the attention is more likely to be caught by them. There is nothing abnormal in the condition, except perhaps that the eye should not be kept staring at bright, featureless surfaces.

Floating specks and the shadows of blood cells probably account for many of the alarming stories which, beginning in the U.S.A. during the summer of 1947, described mysterious objects " moving at over 1,000 m.p.h.," and seen in the sky by observers in many parts of the world. These were variously described as " airships," " flying flapjacks " and " saucers in formation."

The visual disturbances which accompany certain types of acute headache are in quite a different category, since the actual organ involved in this case is the brain. Any drastic alteration of the pressures in the blood-vessels of the brain, or the presence of certain toxins, may stimulate or benumb the nerve cells, producing impressions of sudden darkness, or of flashes of light.

Retinal Trouble

Serious breakdown of the retina may develop gradually or suddenly, although in the latter case there is nearly always some sign of physical distress or an obvious state of general ill-health as a preliminary. The sensitivity of a particular area of the retina may be lost completely—*scotoma*—or the retina as a whole may become less sensitive. When part of the retina is affected it is usually only in one eye. Occasionally the area of most acute vision is involved—a condition termed central scotoma. The person is unable to see an object when the eye is directed straight at it, but can see fairly well the surrounding objects. Such a small blind patch may develop in any part of the retina, and the direct cause is commonly an inflammation in the optic nerve. Here again, the importance of blood composition is obviously paramount.

Sometimes there is a loss of function in the outer regions of the retina—usually of both eyes simultaneously —so that the person can see little outside the small area directly in the line of sight. The effect is described as " tunnel vision," and the impression is similar to that of looking through a long dark tube. Localised blind patches are typical of migraine headaches, and there may be temporary tunnel vision which is usually characterised by jagged " edges," and luminous flashes. Permanent tunnel vision imposes much more serious handicaps on the individual than one might expect. There is no broad field of semi-sharp vision, and it is extremely tiring and difficult for the person to locate objects and to avoid collisions when moving about. Anyone who notices a narrowing of his field of vision should take it as a clear warning that it is time to take really drastic action to improve not only his eyesight but the state of his bodily health.

The field of vision can be roughly tested by fixing each eye in turn on some object directly in front, and then slowly swinging the hand, with arm extended, from straight ahead to each side, followed by similar movements upwards and downwards. (Keeping a finger wriggling makes it easier to decide when the hand actually passes beyond the limits of the visual field.) With most people it is normal for the hand to be visible to almost right angles in each direction. (The nose and the eye-brows usually limit the field above and to the inner side.) If your field of vision proves to be less than this, however, and there is no particular discomfort in the eyeballs, there is no cause for immediate alarm. It is only if a similar test some weeks or months later show a further restriction in field, or if the eye becomes painful, that one need be seriously concerned.

The most likely explanation of such a " fade-out " is that a devitalised system finds it impossible to maintain the entire retina in full working order and is forced to sacrifice the outer fringe so that the more immediately essential central area may be kept working. A somewhat similar solution is arrived at in cold weather in individuals with poor circulation. The fingers and toes —the outlying members—become cold and numb, almost lifeless, while the active circulation continues fairly adequately in the central vital organs. It is not possible to say whether the full function of the retina can be regained in any particular case, but certainly it is essential to encourage a more healthy state so that further degeneration may be avoided. The exact forms of treatment and correction called for are usually a matter for professional consideration.

Glaucoma

Loss of peripheral vision is sometimes associated with a very acute and distressing condition—*glaucoma*. In this the pressure of the fluids within the eyeball is greatly excessive ; in advanced cases the cornea may be visibly distended, and pain is intense. The condition is often closely related to high blood pressure, and most probably results from an over-consumption of liquids, particularly tea, coffee and alcoholic drinks, and of the acid-forming foods—sugars, starches and proteins. To the touch, the eyeball is board-hard, instead of having its normal " finger-tip " texture. The excess pressure prevents the proper circulation of nutrient fluids within the structures of the eyeball, and this nutritional failure is probably the direct cause of the restricted vision.

In such cases, any attempt to produce improvement by local exercise is worse than futile. Professional advice should be sought before attempting any sort of home treatment—other than the common sense steps of discontinuing such obvious dietary errors as those·listed above.

To keep the outlying regions of a more normal retina alert, one can play little games, such as trying to make out the shape and detail of various objects without looking directly at them. Fix the eye in turn on various points on a wide circle around the object, while keeping the attention on the object. (That the point of attention and the line of acute vision need not coincide may be a discovery to some. The more crafty, however, will know full well that they can keep their eyes fixed on something straight ahead while all the time watching very alertly what is going on at right angles—" out of the tail of one's eye.")

One should not be aware of any strain during this exercise, which should be done quite effortlessly and freely. Always finish by looking directly at the object, so that the area of acute vision is given its fair play. (It is most desirable that in the ordinary way the eye should be accurately aimed at the object of attention. " Laziness " in this respect can lead to severe headaches and other signs of strain and inefficiency.)

Detachment of Retina

A dramatic type of eye injury is detachment of the retina. This is occasionally produced by violence, but can also result from a long-continued strain. It is found that this accident generally occurs to short-sighted persons. In a healthy body the various parts are well proportioned, and in a state of balance. Accidental jars are absorbed uniformly by the tissues involved, and tearing asunder rarely occurs. In ill-health, however, the mechanical strength of the tissues is lessened, and abnormal and uneven strains increase the chance of serious damage. Apart from obvious shock, it has been suggested that detachment may result from the retina attempting to move forward into the focal plane, where the eye has either become elongated or the lens is over-convex. Whether that suggestion is valid or not—it is certainly logical and reasonable [1]—there can be no questioning that the condition is more likely to occur in general ill-health and short-sightedness.

[1] For further observations on the intelligence and adaptive ability of the body cells, see *Why Not Smoke?*

The usual symptom of detached retina is a sudden indistinctness and possibly darkening of part of the field of one eye. If this occurs the person should immediately lie down quietly, on the back, so that gravity may assist in restoring the detached tissues to their right position. Quite apart from being the best treatment for the injury, this procedure will minimise the possibility of the other retina following suit. The extreme combination of stresses and strains which caused the first detachment will in all probability ease away within a few days, or even hours, but it is wise to take every precaution against further damage.

Spontaneous re-attachment of the retina occurs in a fair proportion of cases, and the more prompt the treatment, and the more intelligent the patient's behaviour, the better the chance of complete restoration to normal. It is imperative that the patient should immediately undergo a physiological rest, *i.e.*, restrict his diet—preferably taking no food for at least 24 hours —and cut all liquids to a minimum. These, of course, are the conditions we recommend for rapid healing of injury anywhere in the body, but particularly in cases such as this where pressures of fluids and nervous tension play so large a part.

Gentle head movements may assist healing by improving the circulation, and deep breathing will both activate the blood and produce a relaxation of nervous tensions.

The steady, slow rhythm of deep breathing has a quietening effect upon the whole nervous system. Meanwhile, the elimination of waste gases is carried out more efficiently and the intake of oxygen improved.

An allied condition is rupture of a small blood-vessel on the surface of the retina. When this occurs

Y.S.—3

the individual is suddenly aware of a red patch in the field of vision, which usually spreads rapidly and may entirely obscure the sight of the affected eye. Here, too, the predisposing causes are general ill-health combined with severe strain. Unless there has been some accidental injury of the retina—*e.g.*, by intense radiation of ultra-violet or infra-red light—the bursting of a vessel in the eye is comparable with stroke—a hæmorrhage in the brain. In each case, the tissue-quality of the individual has almost certainly been reduced below normal—for example, by established bad habits such as the intake of liquids in excess—and the blood-vessels within the area have become congested. The pressure may be high throughout the body, as in those who habitually overeat of proteins and starches, and who drink or worry excessively, or it may be a local physical condition resulting from tense neck-muscles. The exact differentiation, however, is of little practical importance, since generalised and localised hyper-tensions are but varying individual reactions to the same kinds of errors in living. The escaped blood will normally be readily re-absorbed : but, once more, the cleaner the bloodstream and the more vigorous the circulation, the more rapid and complete the repair.

CHAPTER VI

MINOR DISCOMFORTS AND ACCIDENTS

WE have now dealt with most of the structures of the eye concerned with vision and reviewed their commoner defects and mis-functionings. There remain to be considered some abnormal conditions which, however, are without direct effect on the sight. The " eye," as thought of by most people, is more than the eyeball alone, and conditions involving the lids and the tear-apparatus are usually termed " eye troubles." Foreign bodies " in the eye " rarely penetrate the actual eyeball. Far more commonly they simply lie between the eyeball and the upper or lower lid.

Most pieces of grit or other small particles will find their own way out of the eye, helped by a copious flow of tears. Although there is an almost irresistible inclination to rub the eye, it is probably the worst possible treatment, as it tends to embed the particle in the tissues. Gentle rubbing at a point away from the particle, however, can often help, but perhaps the safest movement is rapid blinking. If the foreign body refuses to leave, it can usually be coaxed out by the individual without even using a mirror. The particle is nearly always under the upper lid, and can in most cases be dislodged by the following procedure : Place the forefinger on the front of the lid, press gently downwards, and at the same time grip the lashes with the thumb. Pull the lid down and out, and then allow it to slip back into place over the lower lid. The lower lid and lashes act as a brush, and unless the particle is really embedded, two or three repetitions of the process will bring it out. Eyelashes can be rather obstinate objects, but if the eye is rapidly blinked they usually " flow " out in a few moments.

If you are trying to remove grit from someone else's eye, or—using a mirror—from your own, the upper lid should be rolled up over a finger or pencil, so that the under surface is visible. If the particle is on the front of the eye, it will be found almost impossible to remove it without causing violent twitching. It is usually worth lowering the lid for a moment, and then re-opening, as the particle may transfer to the inner surface of the lid, which is much less sensitive. The same applies to the lower lid, which can often be manipulated to " pick " the object off the eye, and it is then a simple matter to wipe the lid. To remove the particle, the corner of a clean handkerchief is best, used very carefully. (It is usually less irritating if softened and moistened by biting it first. Don't worry about stray germs—the tears will take care of them.)

If the object is embedded either in the eyeball or the lid, and is something in the nature of a glass or metal splinter, then immediate expert assistance is essential.

A foreign body must either strike the eye with great force, or possess very sharp points or edges if it is to break into the tough outer coat of the eyeball. Corrosive substances, however, can inflict rapid and sometimes permanent injury on the eye. (The immediate treatment is bathing with copious amounts of cold or tepid water.) Damage to the eyeball is particularly grave when it affects the cornea (the transparent part of the sclera or tough outer coat) in front of the eye. Obviously, anything which renders the cornea less transparent or which distorts its perfect curve, will cause some loss of visual acuity. Fortunately, the eye is provided with excellent defence mechanisms which come into action when danger threatens. The first of these is the blink, which occurs whenever the eyelashes are touched, or when there is a sudden or unexpected movement or noise nearby. The closed lids are strong enough to withstand almost any ordinary small missile, and in the course of a year the average eye is probably protected in this way from many hundreds of painful or injurious contacts with dust particles, sand-grains, flies and other objects.

The Need for Alertness

Among children—and some adults—there is a belief that blinking when surprised is a sign of cowardice or timidity. " I made you blink " is a common taunt, but the victim's shame is quite unnecessary. His responses are normal and healthy and it would be a great pity if he succeeded in overcoming the protective reaction.

As a further safeguard, although not quite so rapid in action, the eyeball rotates upward behind the closed lid, so that the cornea is no longer in front, but under the protecting ridge of bone behind the eyebrow. This occurs when—for instance—the person expects some sort of explosion, and also in sleep. If any object then pierces the eyelid, the part of the eyeball likely to be damaged is not the vitally important cornea, but the under-surface of the sclera.

Quite apart from violent injury, the cornea must be protected against the tiny specks of dust which occur in even the cleanest of air. It is the duty of the tear-glands to maintain a steady supply of moisture, which flows gently from the upper and outer part of the eyeball, over the front, and then drains into a little canal at the corner of the eye next to the nose. The upper eyelid, by blinking, helps to keep this film of cleansing fluid even and free-flowing. As already mentioned, many people have lost the natural habit of frequent blinking, and as a result suffer from the effects of inadequate flow—dryness and irritation of the eyeball. The drainage canals empty into the nose, and normally the individual is quite unaware of the process in action. In an emotional upset, the tears may flow more freely, and either drain rapidly into the nose or overflow down the face. Frequent sniffing, nose-blowing, or weeping are the usual outward signs of this extra activity.

If the drainage canals are choked, then even the normal flow may be sufficient to produce weeping. The canals are lined with mucous membrane and this can become swollen and actively eliminating just as that of the nose and throat. As the canals are very narrow, the swollen mucosa blocks the opening, and the tears have to overflow externally—hence the bleary eyes of someone with a bad cold.

Although we have spoken of the cornea as being exposed to the air, this is not strictly accurate. There is a very delicate coating, known as the conjunctiva, which covers the front of the eyeball, and also the inner surfaces of the lids. It is transparent over the cornea, but less so over the " white " of the eye. In this part there are numerous tiny blood-vessels of which only a few are normally visible. Collectively, however, they are detectable as either a bluish or very pale pink tinge over the white. A bluish tinge indicates a lack of oxygen, and in a healthy, fair-skinned person, the white of the eye should not appear to have any colour, but should look " clean." The conjunctiva is exceptionally sensitive, and it is really this structure and not the eyeball proper which gives rise to such acute discomfort when a particle of grit or an eyelash gets behind the lid. The sensitivity is protective, since it serves to call into action such defence mechanisms as copious tear-flow and the immediate attention of the individual. If the tolerance were greater it is certain that a great deal more damage would be done to the eyeball by contact with everyday foreign bodies.

The dangers of reduced awareness are recognised by most Nature Cure followers, particularly when it is produced by sedative and hypnotic drugs. The present instance is an example. If the individual is healthy and alert, the automatic protective mechanisms described above will be rapid and effective. The chance of damage to the eye will be correspondingly reduced. If the individual is less healthy, or drugged, his responses are weaker and more sluggish and he is generally disinclined to " bother " about possible injury to his sight.

Two abnormal conditions of the conjunctival blood-vessels may occur. The first is quite common, and is seen when the conjunctiva has been irritated in any way. The vessels dilate, so that the " white " of the eye becomes pink, and many individual vessels may be visible. Heat, cold, crying, irritant dusts and vapours, and foreign bodies can all produce this effect, and the person is usually described as " red eyed." There is no serious significance in the condition, so long as the individual takes the common-sense step of removing the cause. This is not always easy, especially when the cause is someone else's tobacco smoke ! To the sufferer, inflammation of the conjunctiva feels like a stinging dryness or grittiness in the eye. After the cause has been removed, bathing the eyes briefly in cold water may give an immediate relief and accelerate recovery. Exposure of the eyes to dusty or gaseous irritants sometimes produces a delayed discomfort. Typically, if one spends a summer day cycling or motor-cycling—or motoring in a sports car with the windscreen down—the stream of warm dusty air may keep the conjunctiva too dry, despite the best efforts of the tear-glands. There may only be mild discomfort at the time, but at night when one closes the eyes to sleep, the irritated conjunctiva finds the contact of the eyelids almost intolerable. The situation can be extremely distressing but can be easily prevented by wearing goggles or sun-spectacles.

More dramatic than the foregoing is conjunctival haemorrhage : and indeed it usually indicates a much more serious condition. It may result from direct injury such as a blow to the eyeball, but more commonly it occurs without obvious external cause. The person may awake in the morning with the condition. The white of the eye shows a deep red colour, usually confined to one segment, and not extending over the cornea. If there has been no direct injury, the event indicates that the blood-vessels have been subjected to a greater strain than they can stand. It is likely that a similar dangerous over-strain exists in other parts of the body, most probably within the head. The rupture may have been caused by sudden increase in blood-pressure, or by a gradual loss of elasticity in the vessels—or possibly a combination of both.

In any case, the safest course is to avoid a repetition of anything which might have produced the extra strain, and to try to live a more healthful life in general. So far as the actual haemorrhage is concerned, probably the best treatment is to do nothing at all. It should heal rapidly and clear up within a few days. In the case of known accidental injury cold bathing of the eye may aid recovery, but otherwise it is much safer not to interfere in any way.

A more common condition of the conjunctiva is one liable to cause needless alarm when it is first noticed by the person. It takes the form of a tiny patch of yellowy or brown granules, like a scum on the surface of the white of the eye. These are specks of fatty tissue, and are very usual in elderly folk. They may increase in size from year to year, but in no case have they been found to interfere with the sight ; that is, they never form over the cornea. Their presence probably indicates that the body as a whole is in a state of less than high-level health, and that the person is taking more food than necessary : but by itself the condition has no particular significance.

" Black eyes " and " dark eyes " as usually spoken of, have really nothing to do with the eyeball. A black eye is a condition affecting the eyelids (which, incidentally, are larger than they appear, as they extend over the whole bony eye-socket, the margins of which can be easily felt with the fingers). It usually results from a blow near the eye, often on the rim of the socket, causing the rupture of a small blood-vessel. The escaping blood seeps into the loose tissues of the lids, and, losing oxygen, it assumes a deep purple colour. This, overlaid by the yellowish pigment of the skin, gives an almost black hue. In time, the escaped blood is reabsorbed into the circulation, and the lids resume their normal colour. The reabsorption can be hastened somewhat by gentle massage *after* the internal bleeding has stopped.

Dark eyes, or " rings round " or " shadows under " the eyes are due to the colour of the blood in the vessels of the lids. Here there is no question of escape of blood, but simply a sluggish, poor quality circulation. The circulation through the lids is normally slower than in other parts of the face, and accordingly lack of oxygen and the presence of clogging wastes are more obviously betrayed. This also explains " bags under the eyes," which occur when there is excessive quantity of watery waste in the blood. The blood tends to throw out this excess into all tissues of the body, but particularly where the circulation is slow and where, as in the present case, the skin is loose. The texture and appearance of the eyelids, then, are suggestive of the condition of the bloodstream. If the lids are smooth and pink, the blood is probably clear and well oxygenated. If the skin is puffy and discoloured, the blood is overloaded with water and lacking in oxygen. Such deductions can be very useful as a check on one's own general health. Your popularity may rapidly wane, however, if you insist on giving free diagnoses to your circle of friends and acquaintances !

Elimination of wastes in the region of the eye is usually a sign of a highly toxic bloodstream. As already mentioned, the body normally protects delicate and valuable organs and tissues from possible injury and only allows elimination of this kind to occur when no alternative exit is available. In the region of the eye there are three tissues which may, in emergency, be called upon to act as eliminating organs. The tear-glands produce a relatively copious flow, and accordingly are rapidly affected by changes in the composition of the bloodstream. When there is much acid waste in the blood, the tears are liable to contain a proportion of irritant material. The person may only be aware of a mild " dryness " or " tiredness " of the eyes during the daytime, but during sleep the waste is likely to accumulate, so that a small amount of catarrhal matter is found on the eyelids on awakening. Occasionally the oil-glands at the roots of the eye-lashes also eliminate greasy waste, which, combined with that from the tear-glands, may form a yellowish, crusty mass on the eye-lids during sleep. Such cases obviously indicate the need for more hygienic living, so that the body is not driven to use accessory means of elimination. Also it is important to cleanse the eyes frequently, so that irritation is minimised. The cold-water plunge described on page 37 is probably the safest method, since this stimulates the face as a whole, and does not produce the localised reactions of an eye-bath.

It is always desirable to avoid local stimulating treatment of the eye or ear when these organs are inflamed, since there is a risk of dangerously overloading the delicate structures.

Only in much more extreme cases is the third tissue —the conjunctiva—called upon to eliminate. When this occurs, the inflammation is usually severe, and the waste may be so toxic that pus formation occurs. This clearly shows that the whole body is in such a poisonous state that any form of local treatment—other than simple cleansing—is both futile and dangerous.

In all three types of elimination just described, the main attention should be paid to the general condition of the patient. Local attention is relatively unimportant.

CHAPTER VII

SUMMARY

At this point, it may be helpful to summarise the points raised and the suggestions given in the foregoing chapters.

The eye is a self-regulating and self-healing organ, and its efficiency depends upon (1) the wholesomeness of the bloodstream, which nourishes and cleanses every cell of the body, and (2) the smooth functioning of the brain and nervous system as a whole. Although the body to some extent appears to favour the eye, when there is need to do so, it is impossible for the eyesight to be really efficient if the general health is unsatisfactory. Many drugs, and not least tobacco, can seriously impair the general efficiency of the eye and its mechanisms, and derange optical precision.

The eye requires to be used and exercised regularly if it is to be kept in first-class condition. Many people harm their eyesight by failing to give the eyes sufficiently varied occupations. If it is necessary to keep the eyes on a particular job for a long time, it is very important to interrupt the fixed gaze at intervals, and provide variety by a momentary focusing on nearer or farther and brighter or darker objects. The tiny muscles of the eye are just as liable to become tired and painful as any other muscle of the body if kept in fixed tension for long periods.

For efficient eyesight, the muscles which direct and adjust the eyeball must be accurately controlled and

76

smoothly operated. Poor nutrition and abnormal strains can combine to break down these controls and so produce such conditions as squint, nystagmus, double vision and astigmatism.

Intellect

The effectiveness of sight depends very greatly on recognition of objects and, since recognition is a function of memory, it follows that anything which impairs the memory is also likely to impair visual efficiency. Poor circulation to the head, and sedative or benumbing drugs are the commonest causes. Apart from their very direct physical connection, the eyes and the brain are closely inter-related in other ways. " Vision " is as much intellect as eyesight.

To compensate for the lack of natural exercise under urban and indoor conditions, there are a number of simple remedial movements which can be performed at any time. These are principally designed to bring into action the three muscle groups which are respectively responsible for directing the aim of the eyeball, for regulating the intensity of light on the retina, and for producing sharp focus. Looking at far and near objects in rapid succession, exposing the eyes momentarily to very bright light, and rolling the eyes to follow a wide imaginary circle are typical exercises. For relaxation, Bates' technique of " palming " is particularly helpful. All movements of the eyeball itself and of the surrounding tissues tend to produce a more copious circulation in the region, and keep the tissues of the eye in a well-nourished state. Cold water applications are valuable to the same end.

The eyeball and its inner structures can be deformed in a number of ways, producing characteristic defects of vision of which the most common are short-sight, long-sight and astigmatism. In any particular case the immediate cause may be either in the eyeball, which may be flattened, shortened or elongated, or in a similar deformation of the lens. The deeper cause is usually either an abnormal composition of the fluids in the eyeball or some external strain. The eyeball can be pressed forward by excess fatty and other tissues behind the ball, and it can be pulled out of shape by uneven tensions in the muscles which effect its movement. Even deeper are the nutritional defects and nervous and emotional strains which are the commonest primary causes.

Although an external compensation for many such abnormalities can be provided by the spectacle-lens, this is in no sense a cure for the condition. Indeed the tendency is for the use of spectacles to fix the abnormality, and make it less amenable to remedy by natural methods. Apart from its unfortunate effect on the focusing mechanism, the spectacle-lens has the further disadvantage of restricting the movement of the eyeball in its socket, so depriving it of useful exercise.

Cautionary

The transparency of the internal structures of the eye can be reduced by the presence of toxic matter in the blood, which can in time coarsen the tissues. The same toxic wastes can upset optical perfection by producing abnormal pressures within the eyeball. Excessive heat can be similarly damaging. Reduction of liquid intake (especially tea) and the acid-producing foods (e.g. starches and proteins), and avoiding over-exposure to intense light and heat are elementary steps for avoidance of such conditions, and in attempting their remedy.

The retina itself may be less sensitive to light than normal, either as the result of fatigue or of nutritional failure. In both cases there is a retention of wastes in the sensitive cells, and an inadequate supply of fresh material. In some cases so simple a step as including a few fresh vegetables in the diet may produce marked improvement. In others it is necessary to rectify long-standing errors in posture, breathing and feeding, in which matters skilled attention may be very desirable.

In many circumstances, the eyes are exposed to strains which may be realised only after considerable damage has been done. Ultra-violet light, at high altitudes or in highly reflective surroundings, or from electric arcs, may burn the delicate tissues of the eye and produce very painful damage. Radiant heat can be almost equally insidious, although the individual is at least aware of its presence. Protection in the form of sunglasses and goggles may be essential in such unusual cases. It is also true that many people do their eyes more harm than good by wearing sunspecs.

" Spots before the eyes " and similar interferences with vision may be due either to the presence of impurities in the bloodstream (frequently resulting from overwork or sluggishness of the liver), or simply to the presence of actual particles either within the eyeball or on the surface of the cornea. In the last-mentioned case, very often all that is required is more efficient blinking so that the cornea is kept clean by an adequate flow of tears.

Vision may be defective or absent in certain areas, or the field of vision may be restricted. These defects may be the result of nutritional failure in the retina, or to accidental damage. Restriction of field may be a symptom of excessive pressures within the eyeball, of intense shock or other distress within the brain, often as a result of drugging or operation.

Where the retina has become detached as the result of a combination of ill-health and accidental violence, re-attachment is often possible, but the chance of success is very dependent upon the promptness of the treatment and the full physical and mental co-operation of the patient.

On the outside of the eyeball is the conjunctiva, which covers the front of the cornea and the inner surface of the eyelids. A very sensitive structure, it is readily inflamed by many external irritants. It can also be inflamed by toxins in the blood, or in the tears which flow over its surface. The normal cleansing action of the tears can be helped by a daily plunge of the face into cold water, opening and rolling the eyes while submerged.

The eye has several very effective protective devices, and it is an indication of health if these come into instantaneous action when the occasion arises. Conversely, a sluggish reaction is indicative of poor nervous tone, poor nutrition, or the effect of benumbing drugs.

The cure of " poor nutrition " calls for much more than simply getting the right foods, although that is an essential preliminary. It also involves building up an efficient digestion and an efficient circulation. Healthy blood not only contains an abundance of the various substances required by the cells of the body—including oxygen—but it is free-flowing and richly alkaline, so that acid wastes are readily absorbed, oxidised, and carried off for excretion.

Although orthodox medicine makes much of the fact that " Vitamin A " is essential for eyesight, and points out that carrots are a good source of supply, the sufferer from defective vision should not rest satisfied when he makes carrots an essential part of his diet. Nor even ought he to take unusually large amounts of these or other foods known to contain that vitamin. His aim ought to be to provide his system with a reasonably well-balanced diet, containing a generous proportion of fresh fruits and vegetables, and a minimum of predominantly starchy or watery foods. He must chew his food properly, and encourage his digestion to make the best possible use of it, by keeping food-combinations at each meal fairly simple, and not interfering with digestion by using condiments, tea, coffee or tobacco, or even by strenuous work or exercise too soon after a substantial meal. Remember, too, that oxygen is just as essential as the other nutrients, and that the best blood in the world cannot help the eyes if it is prevented by tension in the muscles in the neck from circulating freely through all parts of the head. There is no such thing as a special diet for patients with eye disorders. If the general diet is satisfactory, and the digestion and circulation are efficient, the body is quite capable of supplying the eyes with all the materials they require, both for maintenance and, where necessary, for repair.

Exercises for improving the posture and general health, and the question of diet are discussed in the final chapters of this book.

CHAPTER VIII

GENERAL EXERCISE

In addition to movements which directly involve the eyes, there are a number of more general exercises which may have an indirectly beneficial effect on these organs.

The principal regions of the body in which muscular weakness, imbalance or strain can affect the general health are : (1) the abdomen, (2) the ribs, and (3) the neck. In addition, the habitual posture is important, since stooping or other forward curvature may aggravate distress in any of these areas.

The Abdomen is contained by a muscular wall, one important function of which is the support which it gives the intestines and other organs of digestion. When the abdominal muscles are in good tone, they help to prevent sagging of the internal organs, and at the same time maintain an appreciable pressure within the abdomen.

When the muscles are in poor condition, they allow the abdomen to sag and protrude, and the internal pressure is low. Both of these results have their effect upon the sense organs within the head. Sagged, distended intestines are sluggish and inefficient : digestion is slow, incomplete and accompanied by much fermentation and putrefaction. This means that the body is unable to extract full value from the food passing through the bowel, and at the same time the blood is liable to absorb considerable amounts of toxic matter. Unless the liver and other blood-cleansing organs are exceptionally vigorous, some of these toxins will reach the eyes and may cause interference with their functions. Since the liver and kidneys are also affected by the sluggish circulation which results from abdominal sagging, other wastes—those normally produced by the tissues of the body—are also liable to be held in the blood for too long and in excessive quantities. Although this is only one probable factor in "spots before the eyes," it can be very important. Even if these symptoms are absent, it is obviously desirable to encourage the most effective and complete action of the digestive and blood-cleansing organs.

When the muscular tone is poor, the blood-vessels within the abdomen are over-dilated. This means that they rapidly become congested—filled with blood which is not replaced with sufficient frequency. This over-congestion of blood, quite apart from its retarding effect on the normal vital activities in the abdomen, is produced most often at the expense of the upper parts of the body. As the abdominal vessels dilate, they fill with blood which would otherwise be kept at a higher level by the pressure in the vessels. The result is that the circulation in the head becomes restricted. When this occurs, the patient may experience a variety of symptoms. If the circulation is slightly diminished, there may only be a tendency to over-rapid tiring of the eyesight, usually coupled with poor concentration and an inefficient memory. (We have noted—*e.g.*, on page 18 —the close connection between vision and other mental activities.)

With more serious restriction of circulation, there may be dizziness and momentary blurring or darkening of the vision—particularly when the person rises suddenly from a sitting position.

In extreme cases of anaemia—or of sluggish circulation—in the head, acute disorders of vision occur. In such cases the brain itself is starved of nourishment and oxygen, and the person's mental distress is made more noticeable by visual and auditory disturbances. But it is not that the head-noises or the visual phantasies produce dementia : all three conditions result from the same cause.

The Ribs ought to be free-moving and raised, so that the chest is active and does not cramp the heart and lungs. In many people the ribs are almost completely rigid and collapsed, so that the internal organs are confined in their movements and local circulation is restricted. When this occurs, both the quantity and the quality of the circulation throughout the body becomes deficient. Active lungs are essential for the efficient oxygenation of the blood, and for the removal of gaseous wastes. If the heart is to work well, and without strain, there must be space for its pulsations to occur free from external pressure or constriction. Quite apart from possible interference with these internal organs, collapsed ribs are rigid ribs and in this state they become, themselves, a direct cause of poor-quality blood. The red blood corpuscles, which are the oxygen-carriers, must be continually replaced as they wear out. The new red corpuscles are produced by the marrow within certain bones of the body. The ribs contain marrow, and the activity of this tissue is affected both by their movements and by the circulation through the ribs. When movement and circulation are free, the marrow is normally supplied, and produces adequate numbers of new cells. When the circulation is restricted, the production of cells is similarly reduced. With many people, particularly those who bend at work over desk or bench, the ribs scarcely move in breathing, the expansion of the lungs being effected solely by the diaphragm. Where this habit of breathing has been established for many years, it may require considerable patience to restore the chest walls to more normal posture and activity.

The Neck, being the flexible connection between the head and body, is a very busy region. The spinal column supports the skull and contains the spinal cord—the great trunk of nerves connecting the brain with all parts of the body. Around the spinal column—" spine " —are various structures, including the blood-vessels which carry blood to and from the head, important nerves, and the muscles which move the head. These vessels, nerves and muscles are closely interwoven, and disturbance in any one can affect the others. Thus we find that if a person is in the habit of holding his head too far forward, the muscles at the back of the neck are in a state of continual tension. This tension tends to constrict the veins which drain used blood from the head, and so produces a congestion within the skull. Congested, stale blood is unable to keep the brain cells and the active tissues of the eyes properly nourished and cleansed, and the result is that very rapidly the efficiency of these organs falls. The person may become irritable, or unable to concentrate or think clearly : his eyes may begin to hurt, or to function unreliably. The muscular tension may also affect the nerves in the vicinity, with rapidly distressing effects on both the digestion and on the heart. Conversely, digestive disturbance, by affecting the nerves, is a common cause of over-strain in the muscles of the neck. " Sick headache " is at least **as**

much due to congestion in the head as to toxic matter in the bloodstream. This type of headache is usually localised " behind the eyes," and produces a tiredness and irritation of the eyes.

Ideally, the head should be held so that it is balanced on top of the spine, without strong continuous muscular effort. Also, the position of the head should be frequently varied, so that each muscle group is given a certain amount of exercise and rest. The almost fixed position when reading, or carrying out intensive close work, is very tiring for the neck muscles, particularly when the head is held forward.

General Posture : There is no necessity to perform a complicated sequence of artificial movements to keep the body in reasonably good shape. A conscious effort to hold the head high is usually a first essential. Brisk walking is probably the best and most useful general exercise. Properly performed it can give adequate play to all the vital regions. If the maximum benefit is to be obtained, it is important to hold one's self erect, to breathe deeply (particularly with the upper part of the chest), to swing the arms freely, and to hold the abdomen " up and in."

In individual cases, however, it may be that one particular area of the body requires special attention. For most people the following simple exercises will be found helpful.

For the Abdominal Region : Ideally the abdominal muscles should be exercised with the body in an inverted position. That is, with the feet higher than the head. In this way the weight of the intestines and other digestive organs is temporarily taken off the abdominal muscles, so that these can contract freely and without strain. (Determined attempts, by persons with sagged abdominal muscles, to exercise them while in an upright position may easily lead to a pressing downward, and so to an unfortunate outcome. By increasing the effects of gravity, they cause still greater congestion and distress in the lower abdomen.) Inverted exercises are intended to contract the muscles to some extent, and so make them better able to support the abdominal contents when the person stands up. To exercise any group of over-stretched muscles, it is essential to make them do heavy work in their most contracted (shortest possible) state.

With the abdominal muscles, one may either fix the body and move the legs, or fix the legs and move the body. In the first instance, no apparatus is required, and very effective exercise can be performed by lying on one's back on some firm surface, lifting the legs, then rolling the body up in the air, so that one is resting only on the back of the head and neck, the arms and shoulders. From this position, the legs may be moved in various directions such as in " striding," " scissors " and " cycling." In striding, one leg is moved forward while the other is moved back, and then their positions reversed. In scissors, the legs are separated sideways, then brought together and crossed, the right leg alter-nately on front of and behind the left. In cycling the feet are circled round as though pedalling a (giant !) cycle.

For abdominal exercise with the legs fixed, some form of apparatus is necessary to hold the feet. It is much better for the body to be tilted, feet high, although considerable benefit can be obtained with a horizontal starting position. The " abdominal board " is a simple apparatus for providing the inclined position, and it need consist only of a plank about 5 feet long, with a leather strap at one end, for the feet to slip under, and a cross-piece at the other, to give steadiness. The strap end is rested on a chair or other convenient object, and the other on the floor. The feet are hooked under the strap, and the head rests on the floor. The arms may be rested, passively, on the abdomen. The body is then raised slowly and steadily until it is at right angles to the legs, and then slowly lowered to the starting position. The movement may be repeated half a dozen times. If the person finds this easy, the exercise may be intensified by placing the hands behind the head. (Usually, however, the individual who can do this has no need to give the abdomen special exercise.)

For the Ribs : Any movement which combines deep breathing with an upward swinging or stretching of the arms will tend to improve the capacity and mobility of the chest. Without apparatus, the arms may be swung forward and upward as the breath is drawn in, until the arms are straight up above the head at full inspiration. Then, without a pause, breathe out while lowering the arms outward to the side, back to the starting position. The breath may be taken in slowly and steadily, and the upward arm movement similarly timed, while for a more vigorous exercise the breath may be rapidly drawn in, as the arms are swung rapidly upward, coming to a stop with a jerk. This latter movement, however, should not be attempted until the slower movement has been thoroughly mastered.

With apparatus, the ribs can be raised and moved by grasping any support above the head, and pulling downward with the arms. The person need not lift himself clear of the ground, although this should be attempted. It is important not to jerk in this movement.

The pull is exerted progressively as the breath is taken in, and relaxed as one breathes out.

For the Neck: Anything which stretches the muscles in turn will help to counteract continued strain (a common condition in desk workers, and organisers in general), and so ease excessive tensions. To ensure fair treatment it is advisable to follow a simple routine, such as the following :—First movement : Press the head *slowly* down and forward as far as it will go, then slowly bring it up and press it back to its limit, repeat slowly and steadily. After a few repetitions, begin to exert a stronger pressure at each end of the movement—which may cause momentary feeling of pain or " burning "—but avoid any jerkiness. In all neck movements, a slow, steadily increasing pull is absolutely essential for relaxation.

Second movement : Keeping the face to the front, press the head down to one shoulder, then over to the other. Repeat as before. (Perform in front of a mirror at first, and make sure that the shoulder is not pulled up to meet the head !)

Third movement : With the head upright, turn the face slowly from left to right and back again, repeating with slowly increasing pull, as before.

Fourth movement : Keeping the face to the front, roll the top of the head in as wide a circle as possible, first clockwise then anti-clockwise. This movement should be slow, as all the others, and if properly performed the nose should only swing up and down—not from side to side. Here again, a mirror will help to achieve the desired strong " grinding " action.

With some people, head exercises of the foregoing kind produce acute dizziness. This really confirms their need for such exercises, although in the early stages the movements should be performed very slowly, and with only two or three repetitions of each. Do the movements sitting if this gives greater confidence and pause for a few seconds if vertigo becomes troublesome.

CHAPTER IX

DIET

As already indicated, any suggestion that health of the eyes is produced by a special diet is quite misleading. Although these organs, with their associated structures, require particular food substances, there is no need whatever to make one's diet abnormally rich in materials known to contain these ingredients. It is known, for example, that if there is insufficient vitamin A in the diet, the eyesight suffers. But little or nothing is to be gained, either prophylactically or remedially, by taking massive quantities of carrots. In *normal* quantities, however, these may contribute considerably to proper and healthful nutrition, which benefits the system as a whole. The human body is highly developed to make almost unbelievably efficient use of all natural foods, when these are presented to it in reasonable variety. It is able to make its selections and maintain a healthful balance in the bloodstream of the essential nutrient, cleansing and structural materials.

Unfortunately, the prevailing tendency in civilised countries is to make foodstuffs of all kinds progressively less natural and wholesome. In order to make possible long-distance transport and long-term storage, many staple foods are processed to remove or destroy their more living parts. Thus we find that mutilated, bleached and adulterated (" white ") flour is almost universal in this country,[1] as is damaged and sterile (" pasteurised ") milk. Canned foods, too, which are little more than fuel plus flavour, form an increasingly large part of the diet. It is not surprising that various deficiency diseases are becoming more evident, and, as we have already noted, deficiencies and lack of balance are likely to show first in the most highly developed organs of the body. The disturbances caused by tea, coffee, tobacco and alcohol may be less immediately obvious to the lay onlooker, but in many cases quite clear to the trained observer. These drugs each have their own characteristic effects, but in general terms they all tend to make digestion and selection of foods less efficient, and interfere with the nutrient and cleansing activities of the bloodstream. They should all be avoided by anyone seeking to improve his general health, mental balance and perception—including eyesight.

If one simple rule were strictly observed, there would be no need whatever for any intensive study of dietetics. *Let all foods be taken as fresh and unaltered as possible.* The natural tastes and selectivities of the body are marvellously equipped to assure a balanced nourishment of the system. But when the tastes of foods are altered—by concentrations, extractions, cooking and added flavourings and seasonings—the natural hungers and appetites become perverted. At the same time, the balance of the materials in the foods is upset.

[1] For approximately half a century virtually all the white flour in this country has been chemically treated to bleach and " mature " it artificially. One medical observer has reported a possible connection between the chalky matter added to flour (on Government orders) and the eye-disorder cataract. The presence of excess mineral calcium in the blood is believed to be one causative factor in the condition.

Nearly always this alteration reduces the amount or availability of the organised minerals and vitamins, while leaving the sugar, starch, fat or protein content little affected. (Cooking, however, can produce profound, and sometimes very unhealthful changes in proteins.) Economic difficulties and political arrangements also have their damaging effect on national habits of eating. Instead of organising a plentiful supply of cheap fresh home-grown grains and vegetables, we find that much of our grain crop is exported as whisky, while unripe fruit and wilted vegetables (to say nothing of tobacco) are imported at relatively high prices. Instead of the small dairyman being encouraged to distribute directly fresh, clean, undamaged milk, we find big combines subsidised to destroy much of the essential goodness, and make inevitable serious delay and decomposition before the milk reaches the consumer. At the same time, the quality of home-grown fruits and vegetables is insidiously undermined by excessive use of artificial fertilisers—again with official approval and, indeed, compulsion.

All this may sound depressingly gloomy, but for the person who is willing to take a little trouble, it is still quite possible to provide his system with a satisfactory diet. In fact, in adopting a food-reform dietary most of the usual changes which must be made consist of omitting or reducing some of the commoner foods and near-foods. When the diet is approximately balanced, health, staying power and full vitality can be built up and maintained on remarkably little quantity. Not immediately, however. The digestive organs must be given time to accustom and re-adapt themselves to normal feeding. Also, since many common drugs have a cumulative and very damaging effect upon the all-important bacterial digestion, time must be given for the body to eliminate any residues of these drugs before normally efficient digestion can be expected. (The subject of digestive efficiency is too broad to be dealt with at all fully here. For a more extensive discussion of this and related matters, see *Intestinal Fitness*, by James C. Thomson and C. Leslie Thomson.)

For most people, the most important points are the following : (1) Eliminate tea, coffee and alcoholic drinks. (*Occasional* small quantities of light wine or cider are unlikely to have any ill-effect, but fortified wines or spirits, or beer in quantity must be barred.)

(2) Reduce all other liquids to a minimum. (There is no need whatever to take " something instead of tea." Tea-drinking is a bad habit, and the substitution of any other unnecessary liquid is only one stage less harmful.) Realise that in temperate climes the body should get all the water it requires in " solid " form—that is, as the normal water-content of fruits, vegetables and, indeed, practically all foods. Drinks taken for their flavour or " refreshing " effect are likely to interfere with digestion, unduly increase the blood-pressure, and overload the kidneys. Far from " flushing out the kidneys," as is popularly imagined, the unnecessary consumption of water, drinks and sloppy foods simply gives the kidneys extra work to do, very often to the detriment of their blood-cleansing activities.

(3) As an extension of the foregoing, all foods should be taken in as dry a form as possible and, where applicable, should be chewy or crunchy rather than soft and sloppy.

(4) Although cooked foods are not ideal, for most folk it is both convenient and reasonable to have one cooked meal in the day.

But remember that cooked food is partly damaged food, and accordingly it is important to make fresh uncooked fruits and vegetables at least the major part of one other meal. (See note (10) for suggested daily menu.) All foods, with the possible exception of flesh, should be well chewed : this applies particularly to uncooked—salad—vegetables, which must be very finely divided in the mouth if the intestinal digestion is to be effective. (Those who complain of indigestion and flatulence after taking salads will usually find a very marked improvement if the quantity is restricted, and extra care is taken with chewing.)

(5) Starchy and sugary foods in nearly every case can be reduced drastically. These include bread, potatoes, milk puddings, porridge, sugar and jams, bakery produce in general and other grains, as rice, oatmeal, breakfast foods. Such cereal foods as are taken should be dry, crisp and whole-grain. Potatoes should be in their jackets. Sugars should be as natural as possible—e.g., honey and dried fruits. Starchy and sugary foods produce much acid waste of a simple type, requiring free respiration for their elimination.

(6) Although a less prevalent error in this country, protein foods are often over-consumed. These include flesh foods of all kinds, cheese and eggs, peas, beans, lentils, nuts and milk. (Milk is an exceptional food, since its water content is actually lower than that of most solid foods : also, in its natural untampered state it contains almost every type of food substance required by the human body—but the proportions are not correct for an adult.) Protein foods produce " heavy " acid wastes which tax the liver and kidneys.

(7) Fatty and oily foods should not normally form a considerable part of the diet. They should be treated

rather as pleasant additions, with a tendency to overwork the liver if taken in excess.

(8) The three foregoing groups of foodstuffs—carbohydrates, proteins and hydrocarbons, to give them their general chemical groupings—should constitute *less than half the total weight* of the diet. The greater part should consist of as wide a variety as possible of fresh vegetables and fruits. Naturally, the variety and types will be limited at certain times of year, and in some localities a good deal of determination may be required to ensure an adequate supply even during the most favourable seasons. So far as practicable, try to obtain fruits and vegetables which are grown locally—and if at all possible, grown on organically fertilised ("composted") soil. The coarser types of vegetable may be cooked, but as already indicated, the greater the uncooked proportion of vegetable the body can be persuaded to digest and utilise, the better. Green leafy vegetables and root vegetables supply generous quantities of organised mineral salts, which are essential for the body's normal handling and excretion of the acid wastes of starch, sugar and protein foods. They also provide a variety of vitamins. Fruits also contain salts and vitamins, and are generally more easily digested than leafy or root vegetables. In temperate climates, however, acid fruits should be treated with respect, as they can have a seriously irritating effect on any part of the body which may happen to be eliminating wastes vigorously. Thus if the person is troubled with inflamed eyes (keratitis, conjunctivitis, blepharitis, etc.), avoid acid fruits at least temporarily, especially those of the citrus group—oranges, lemons, and grapefruits.

(9) Digestion is most efficient when food is taken only two or three times in the day. Drinks, snacks and

sweets taken between meals or before going to bed are all disturbing and totally unnecessary. For many people, a suitable arrangement is to have a very small breakfast, a moderate meal in the middle of the day, and the principal meal in the early evening—that is, after the day's main work is finished.

Mid-day is perhaps the best time for the salad meal, and evening for the cooked meal. However, if the mid-day meal must be hasty, a *small* cooked meal may be preferable, and the more leisurely evening time devoted to a thorough chewing of the salad stuffs.

(10) A suggested typical daily routine is as follows :

Breakfast : *Summertime*—Small mixed salad or one or two pieces of sweet fresh fruit (*e.g.*, an apple and a small bunch of grapes). Fresh and dried fruits may be taken together for variety. *Wintertime*—Small amount of dried fruit—*e.g.*, four prunes, *or* equivalent amount of figs, apricots, peaches, dates or raisins. Slice of brown bread toasted and buttered cold, *or* small quantity of whole-grain breakfast cereal. If drink desired, cup of weak cocoa or dandelion coffee. (The various proprietary cocoas flavoured with malt etc., are quite permissible).

Mid-Day Meal : Fair-sized mixed salad. Basis of green leafy vegetables, as lettuce, cress, watercress, with additions of tomato, carrot, turnip, beetroot (grated raw, or cooked and sliced) celery, radishes, cucumber etc., as available, and to choice. When lettuce is not available, the green leafy bulk may be made up with brussels sprouts, chopped savoy or cabbage. The less dressing taken with salad the better, but a teaspoonful of olive oil and a squeeze of lemon are quite permissible. A wholemeal roll, or a couple of pieces of crispbread, with butter, and a small amount of cheese, honey or home-made jam. Glass of milk.

Evening Meal : Selection of vegetables, *quick*-boiled or steamed. One medium-size or two small potatoes, boiled or baked in their jackets. Alternate days, made-up savoury dish of egg, cheese, nuts, or dried peas or beans. Other days, begin the meal with a good thick soup made from vegetables—*e.g.*, Scotch broth, tomato, celery or onion soup. In place of meat or bone stocks, use rice or barley if desired. For dessert, a piece of fresh sweet fruit, or stewed fresh or dried fruit. Occasionally, a steamed pudding, egg-custard or gelatine dish. Small cup of dandelion coffee if desired.

No other food should be taken between mealtimes, and if chocolate or sugar confectionery is taken, it should be at the end and as part of a meal.

As already suggested, the last two meals may be interchanged if this is more convenient.

The general composition of the diet will inevitably vary from season to season. This is perfectly natural and healthful, and advantage should be taken of better supplies of fresh fruits and vegetables in summer and autumn, which should then take the place of the relatively inert cereals, breadstuffs, potatoes and dried fruits.

The dietary outlined above is intended for an adult living in this country. For children, fresh milk should be taken at two meals, and the amount of proteins such as cheese, eggs, peas, beans and lentils and nuts may be *slightly* increased.

Flesh foods are not recommended, but if these are taken, avoid pork, fish, game, poultry, rabbit and the like. Small quantities of fresh beef, mutton or offal may be substituted for the vegetable proteins.

These dietary suggestions are necessarily very sketchy, and for fuller information the reader is referred to *About Eating for Health* by Bertram T. Fraser, M.A., B.Sc., and the present writer, and to the recipe book *Food for Health*, by J. R. and J. E. Thomson.

INDEX

Abnormalities of vision, 20, 26, 38
Art of Seeing, 24, 29
Astigmatism, 22, 44

Bates, W. H., 23, 29, 30
Black eye, 73
Blind spot, 48
Blinking, 57
Bloodshot eye, 72

Cataract, 46
Colour-blindness, 10
Convergence, 34

Dangers to eyesight, 52
Detachment of retina, 64
Diet, 81, 91
Drug effects, 10, 71, 92

Exercises, eye, 30, 31
Exercises, general, 82
Eye movements, 12, 16, 28
Eye muscles, 16
Eye structure, 13, 16

Focusing abnormalities, 38
Focusing mechanism, 23
Foreign bodies, in eye, 67

Glasses, legitimate use of, 43, 54
Glaucoma, 46, 63
Good Sight Without Glasses, 29

Haemorrhage, conjunctival, 72
Haemorrhage, retinal, 66
Huxley, Aldous, 24, 29
Hypermetropia, 27

Iris defects, 47
Irritation of eye, 67

Lens defects, 26
Lens function, 15, 16, 25
Long sight, 27, 39, 42

Memory and recognition, 18
Myopia, 26, 40

Nerve, optic, 14, 16, 57
Nervous strain and eyesight, 21
Night blindness, 51
Nystagmus, 20

Optic nerve, 14, 16, 57

Palming, 30
Perception, 5, 18
Presbyopia, 27
Protection of eyes, 53, 69, 72

Retina, 49
Retina, defects of, 61
Retina, detachment of, 64
Retina, haemorrhage in, 66

Short sight, 26, 40
Smoking, 10
Spots before eyes, 57
Strabismus, 20
Sun-glasses, 53
" Sunning," 47

Tobacco, 10
Tunnel vision, 61
Toxic effects, 57

Ultra-violet light, 52

Vision, disturbances in, 58
Vision, mechanism of, 16

Water-treatment for eye, 37